Prithvi Raj · Hans Nolte · Michael Stanton-Hicks

Illustrated Manual of Regional Anesthesia

Conception, Realization, Consultation, Organization: Bureaux Bassler, Karlsruhe, FRG
Artist: Wolfgang Rost, Graphic-Design

Part 1: Transparencies 1–28

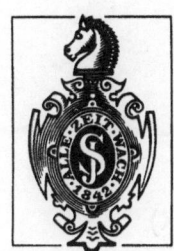

Springer-Verlag Berlin Heidelberg GmbH

ISBN 978-3-642-47799-7   ISBN 978-3-642-61386-9 (eBook)
DOI 10.1007/978-3-642-61386-9

①

②

③

④

① Cervical: 7 vertebrae, 8 spinal nerve segments (C1–C8). ② Thoracic: 12 vertebrae, 12 spinal nerve segments (T1–T12). ③ Lumbar: 5 vertebrae, 5 spinal nerve segments (L1–L5). ④ Sacral: sacrum, 5 spinal nerve segments (S1–S5)

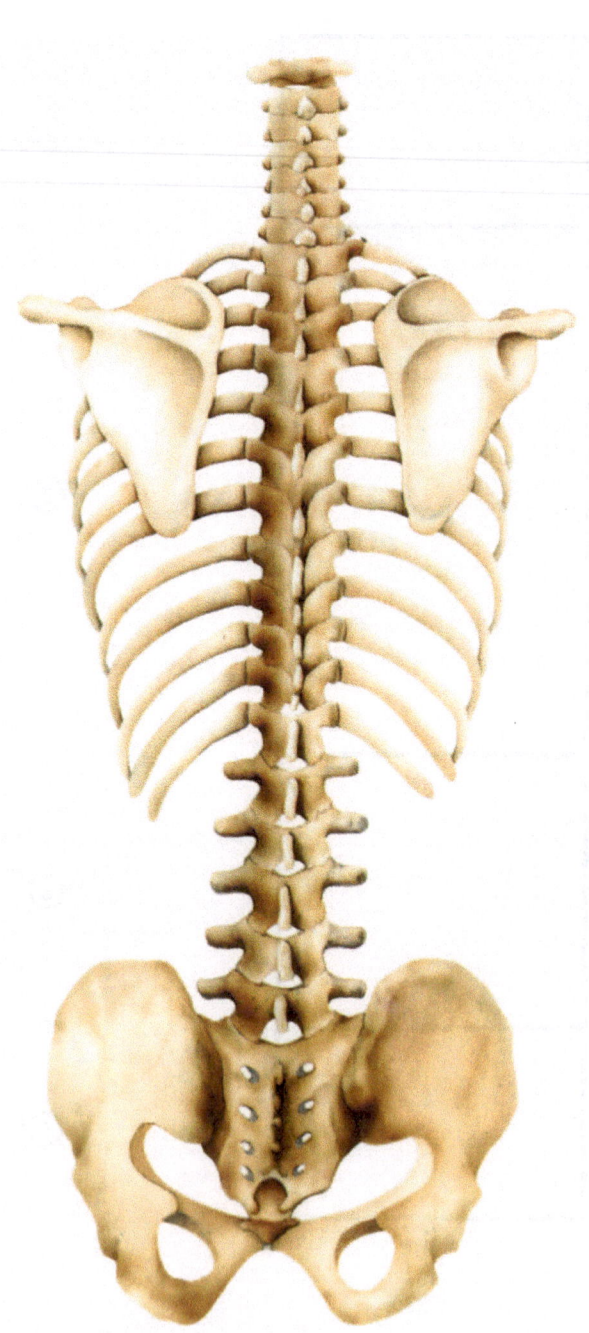

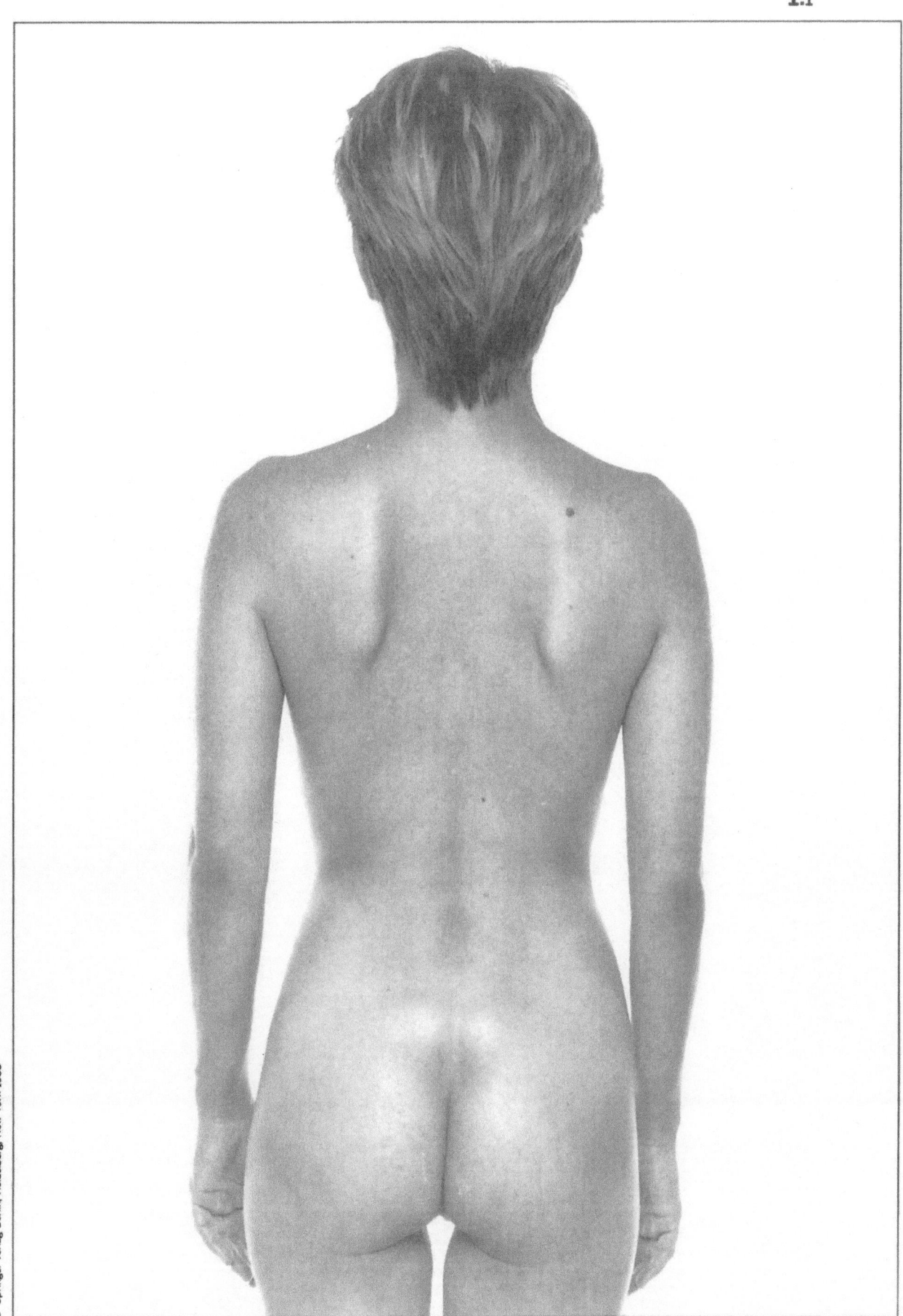

Anatomy of the Spine

1

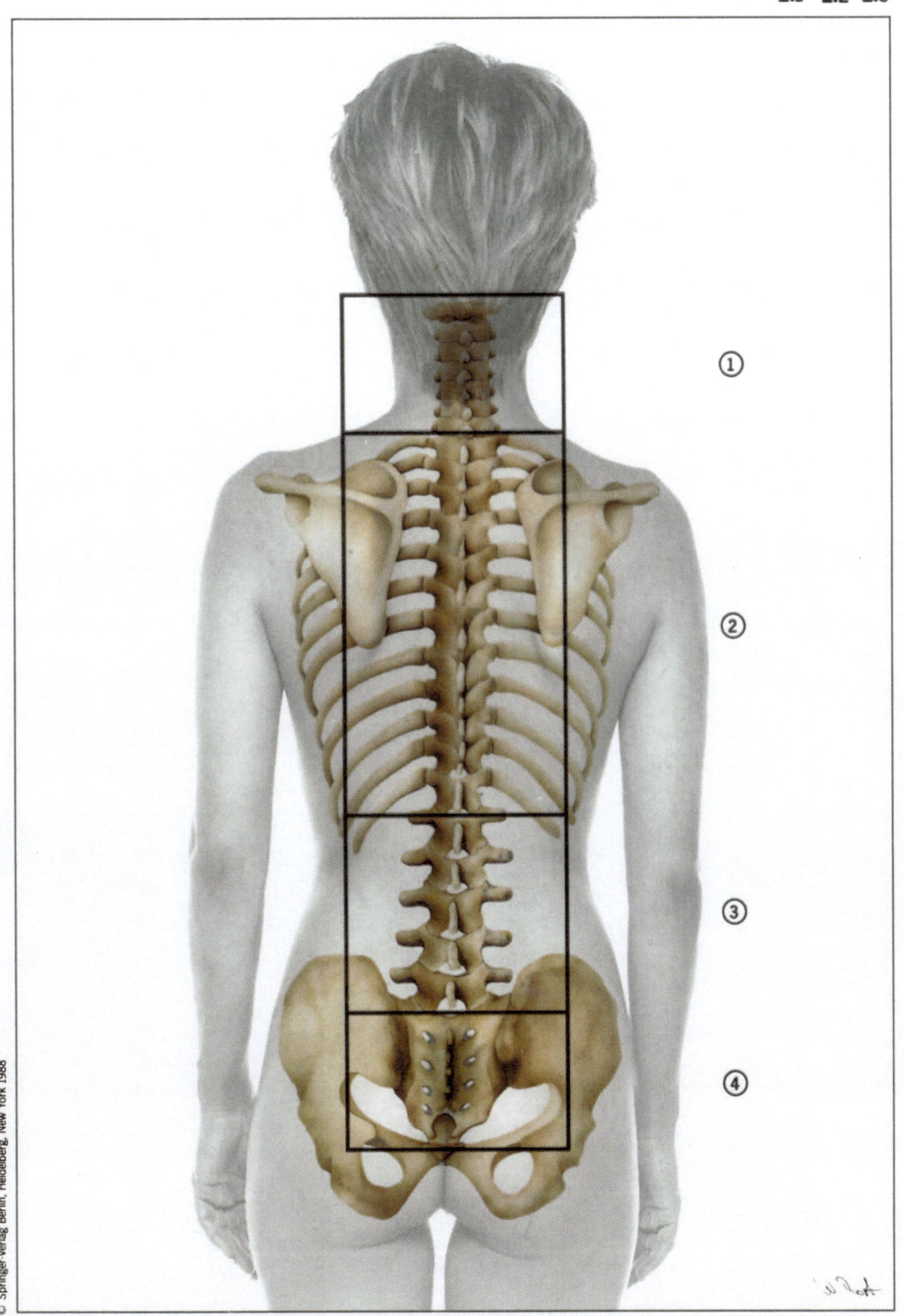

① Cervical: 7 vertebrae, 8 spinal nerve segments (C1–C8). ② Thoracic: 12 vertebrae, 12 spinal nerve segments (T1–T12). ③ Lumbar: 5 vertebrae, 5 spinal nerve segments (L1–L5). ④ Sacral: sacrum, 5 spinal nerve segments (S1–S5)

① Midline approach. ② Paramedian approach. ③ Taylor approach. ① Iliac crest. ② Spinous process of L3. ③ Spinous process of L4. ④ Spinous process of L5. ⑤ Posterior superior iliac spine

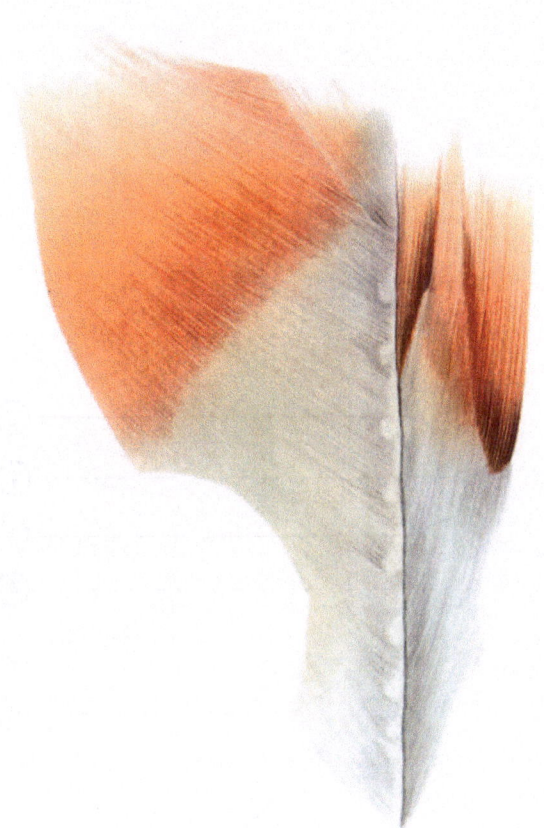

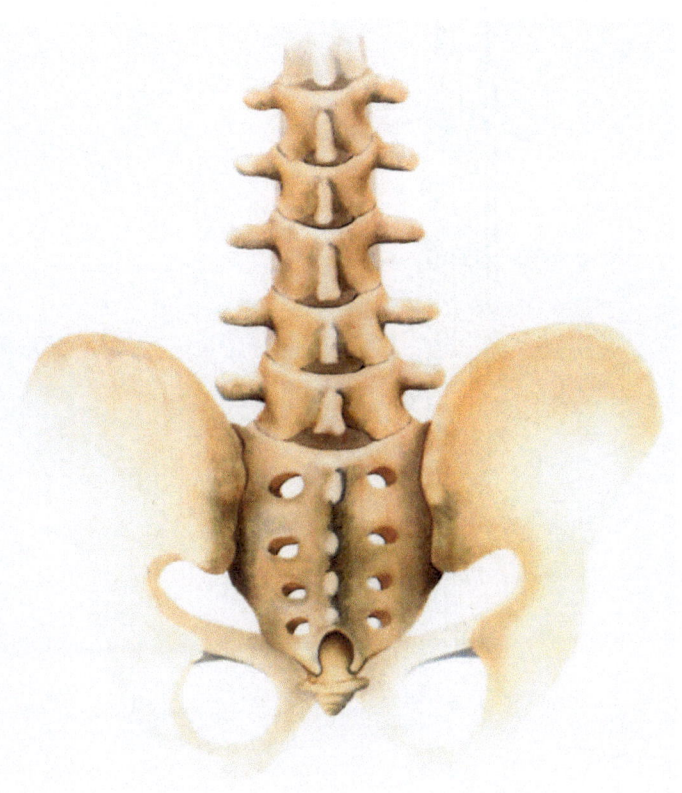

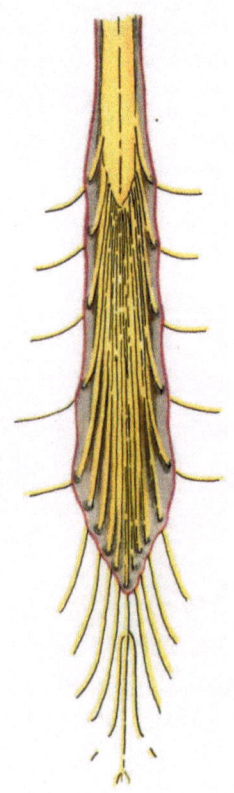

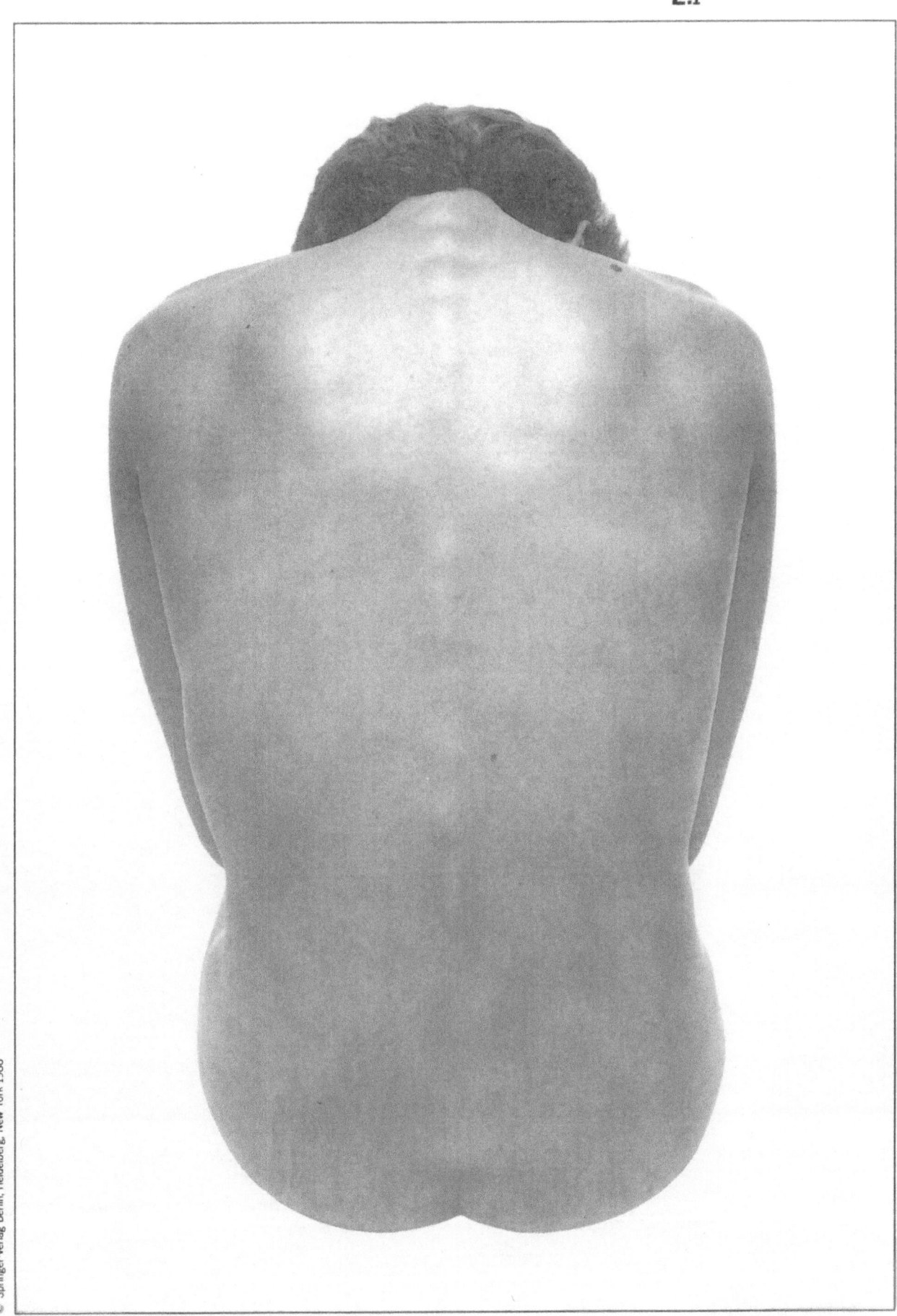

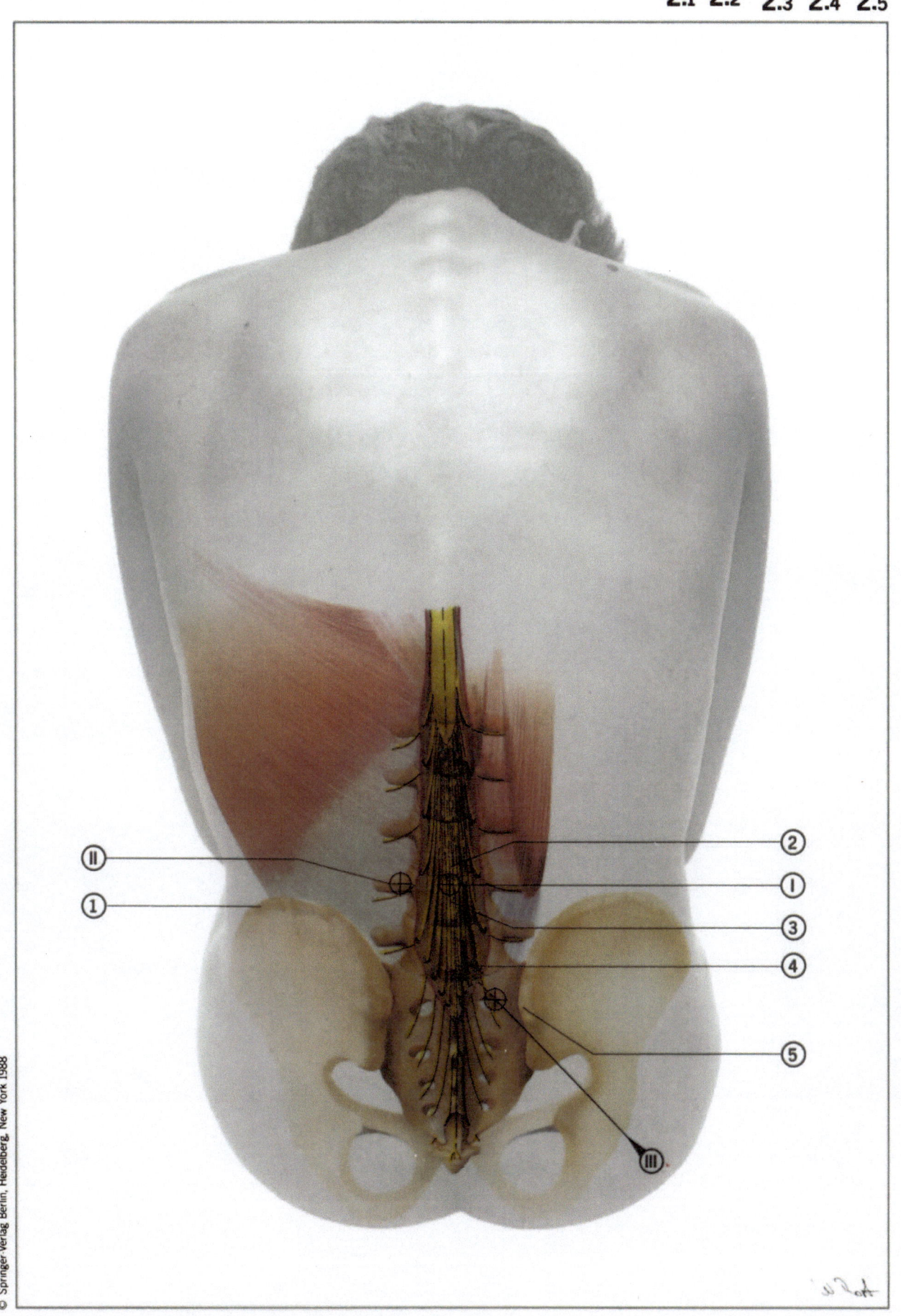

Ⓘ Midline approach. Ⓘ Paramedian approach. Ⓘ Taylor approach. ① Iliac crest. ② Spinous process of L3. ③ Spinous process of L4. ④ Spinous process of L5. ⑤ Posterior superior iliac spine

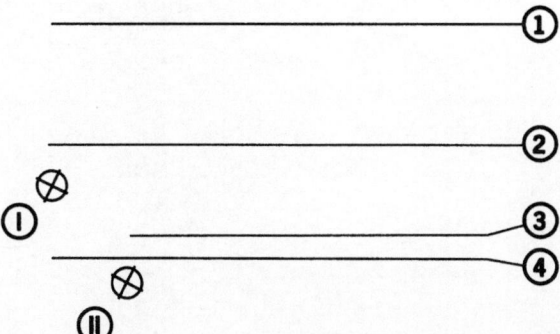

Ⓘ Midline injection site at C7–T1 interspace. Ⓘ Injection site for paramedian approach at inferior border of T1. ① Interspace between spinous processes of C5 and C6. ② Spinous process of C7. ③ Lamina of T1. ④ Spinous process of T1

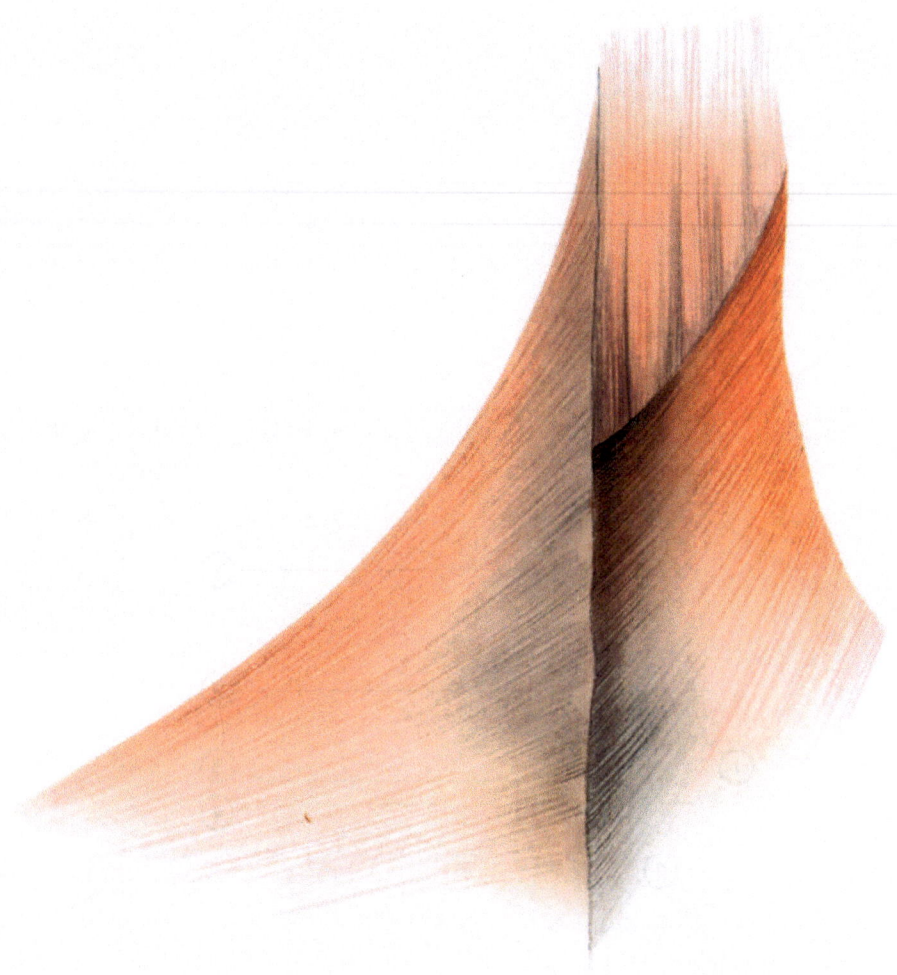

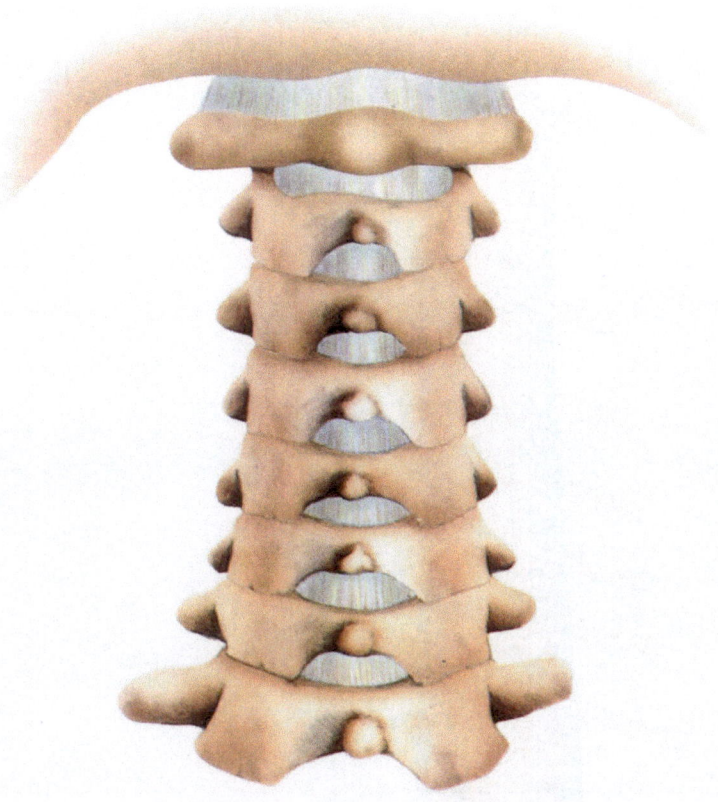

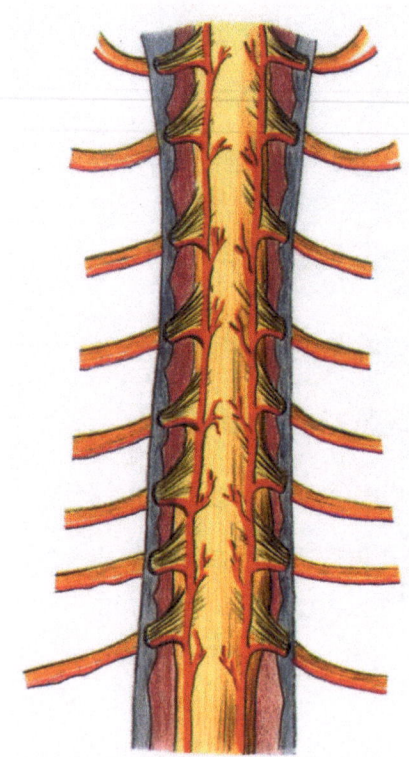

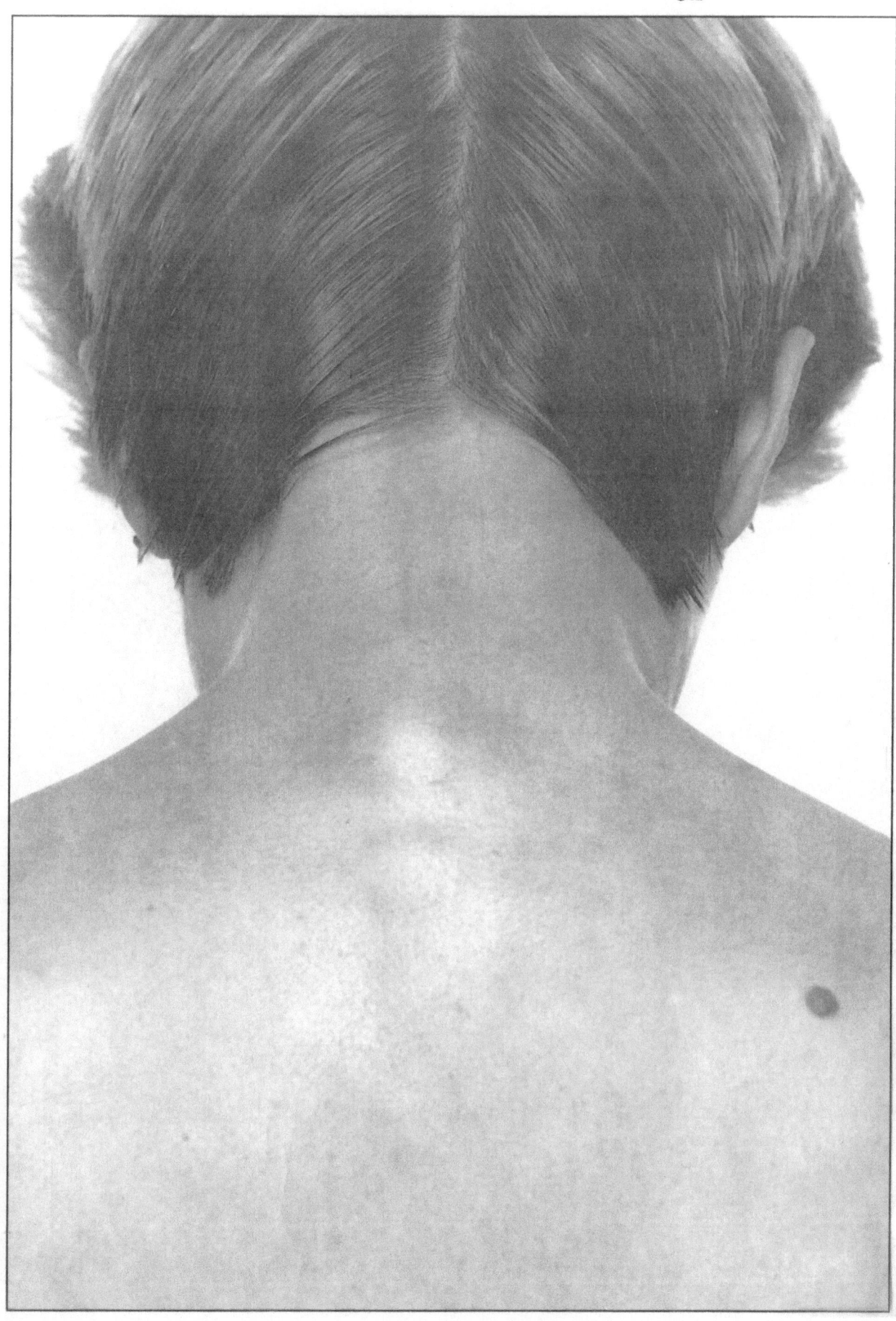

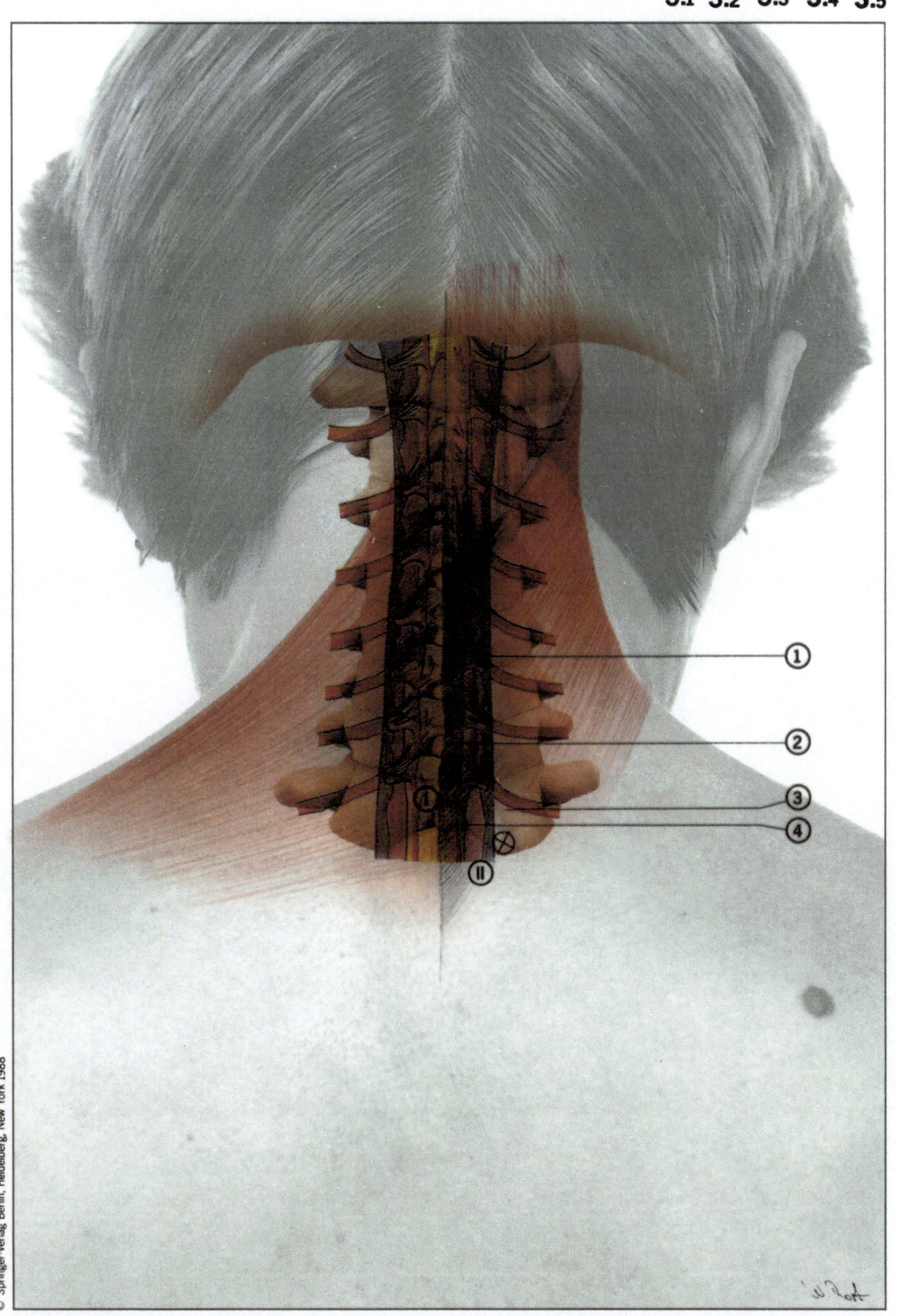

① Midline injection site at C7–T1 interspace. ⑪ Injection site for paramedian approach at inferior border of T1. ① Interspace between spinous processes of C5 and C6. ② Spinous process of C7. ③ Lamina of T1. ④ Spinous process of T1

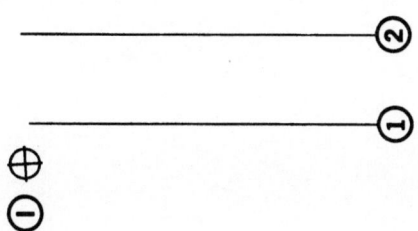

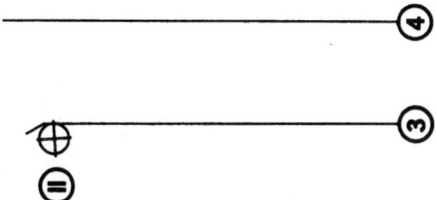

① Midline injection site at T10–T11. ⑪ Injection for paramedian approach at T3–4 interspace. ① Spinous process of T10. ② Spinous process of T9. ③ Spinous process of T3. ④ Spinous process of C7

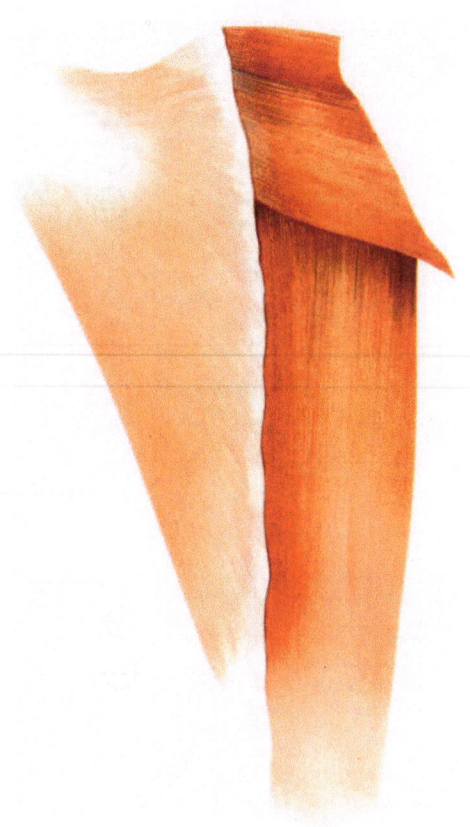

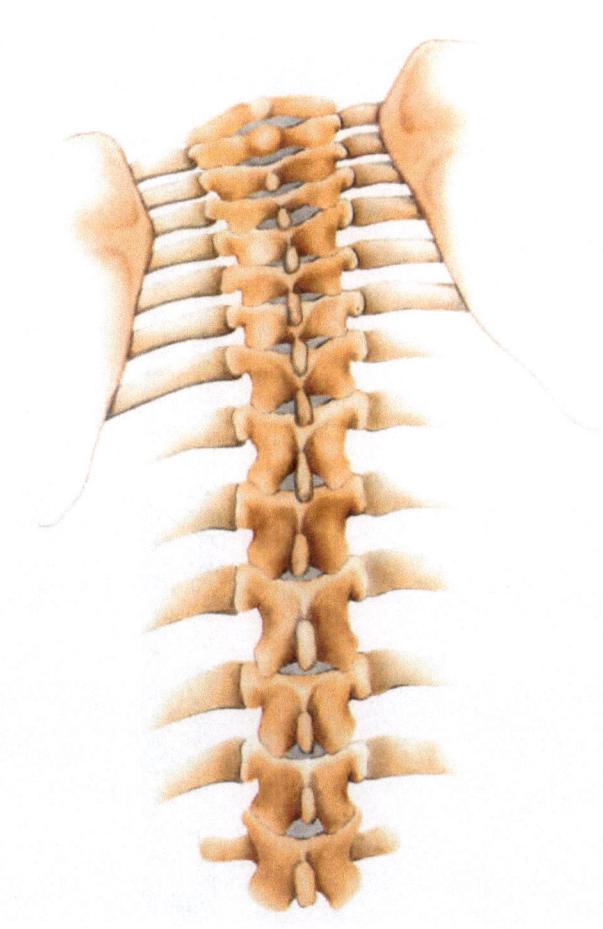

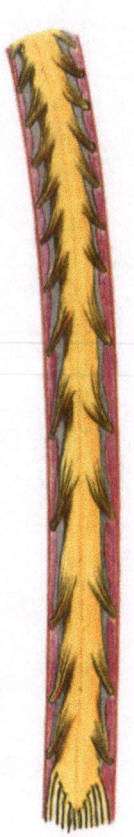

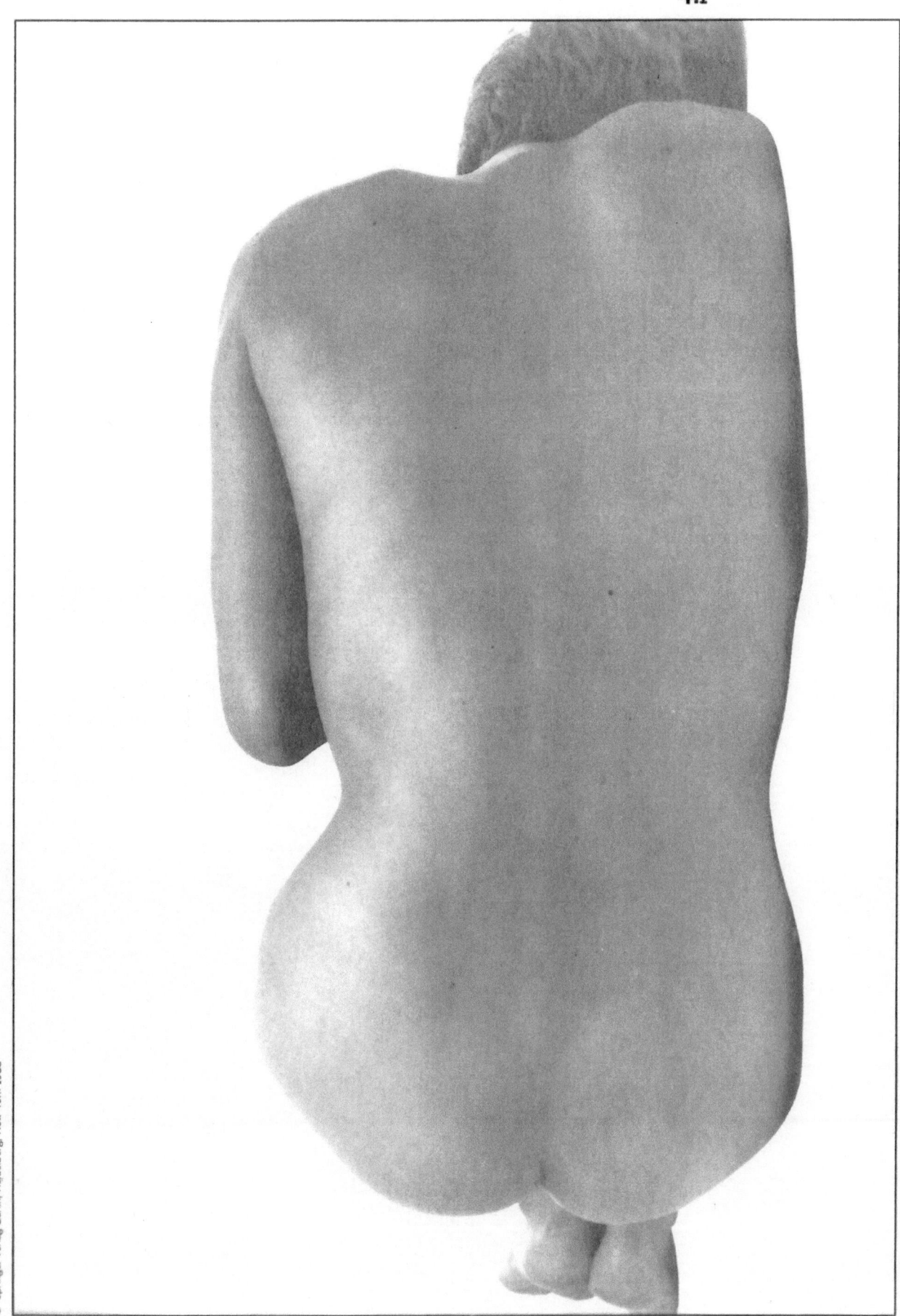

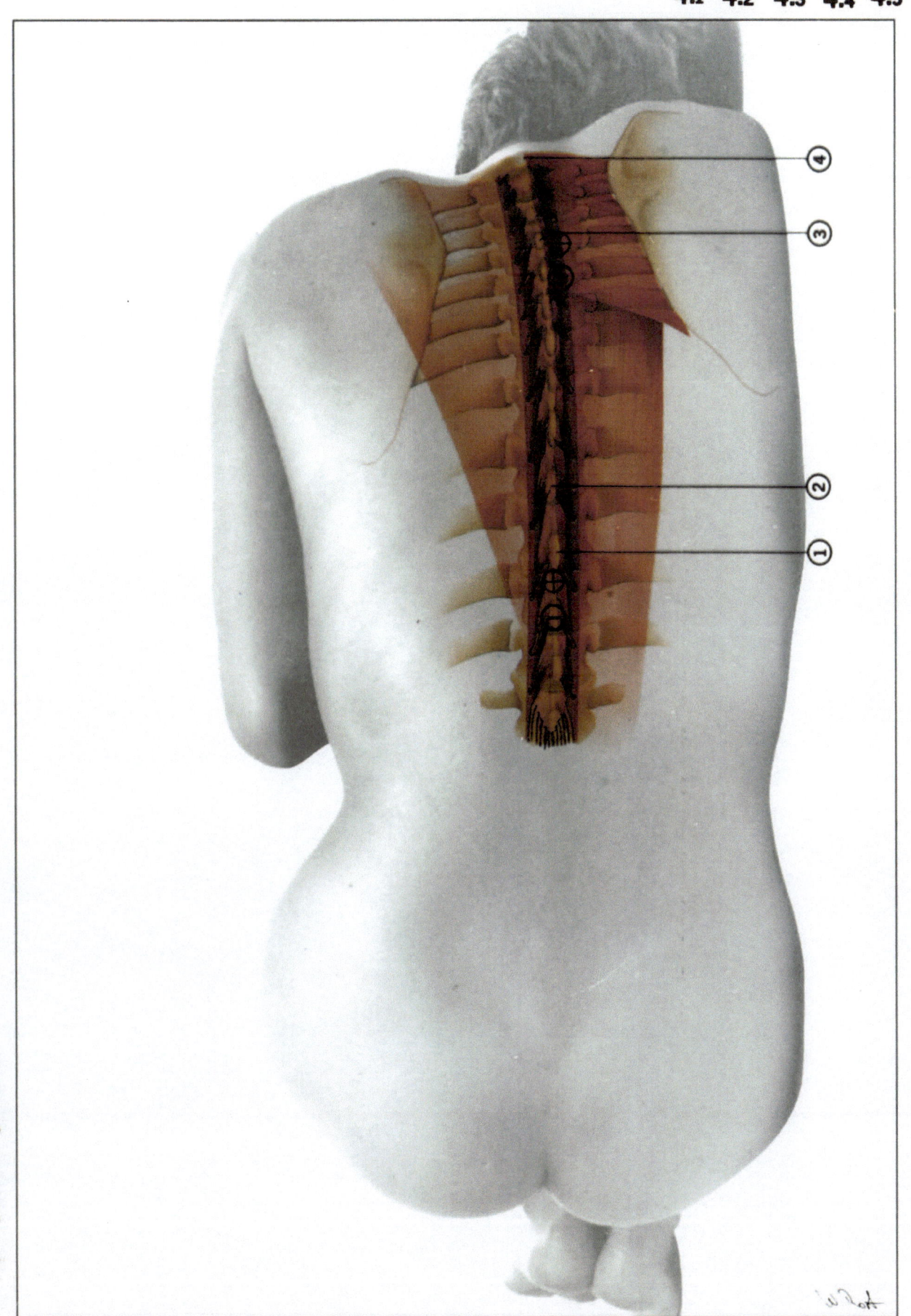

① Midline injection site at T10–T11. ② Injection for paramedian approach at T3–4 interspace. ① Spinous process of T10. ② Spinous process of T9. ③ Spinous process of T3. ④ Spinous process of C7

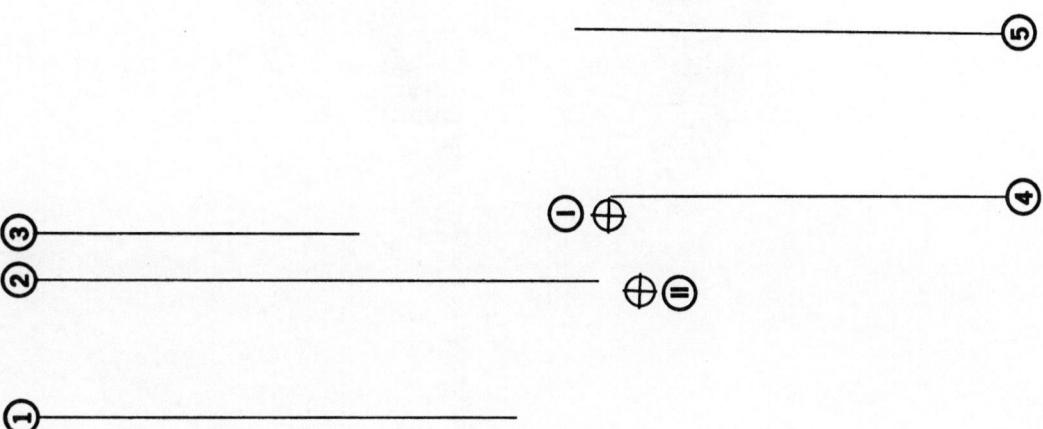

① Injection site for midline approach to L3–4 interspace. ⑪ Injection site for paramedian approach to L3–4 interspace. ① Posterior superior iliac spine. ② Spinous process of L4. ③ Superior iliac crest. ④ Spinous process of L3. ⑤ Lamina of L1

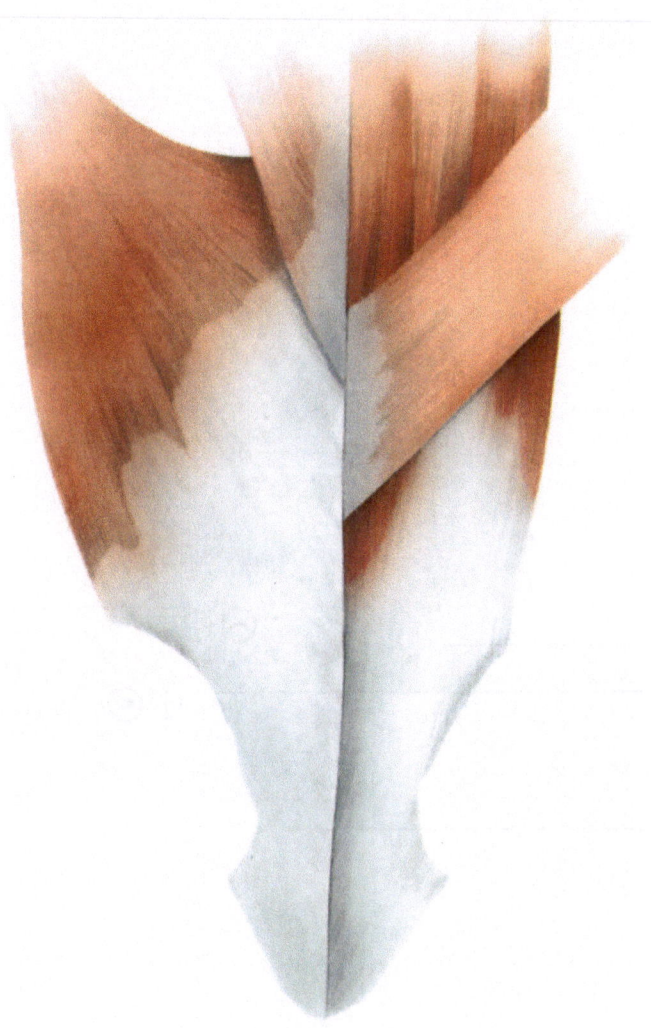

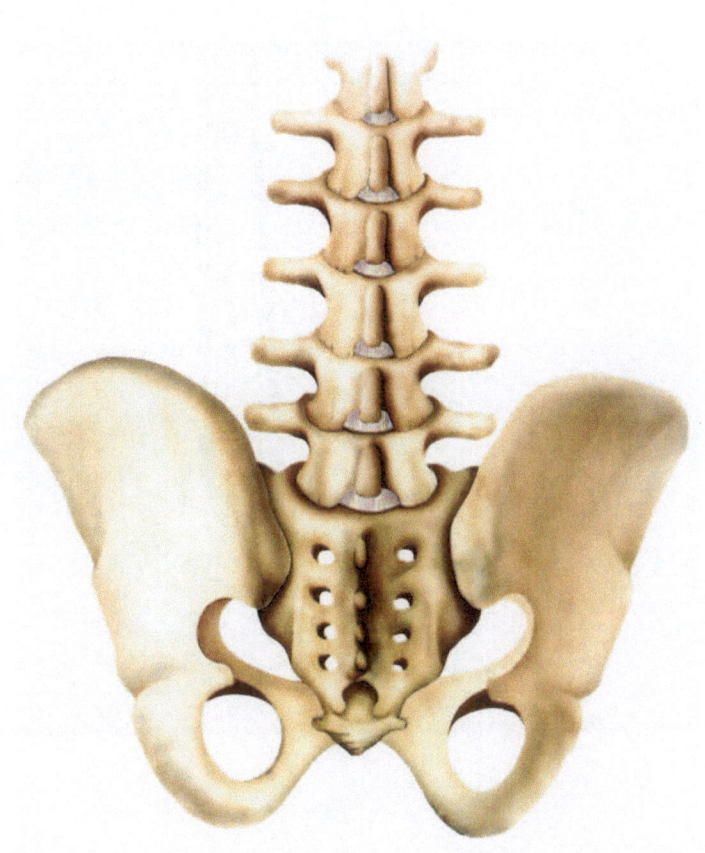

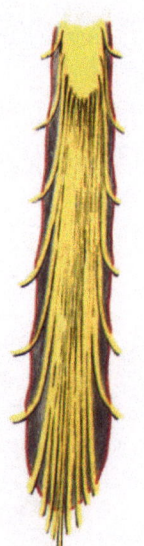

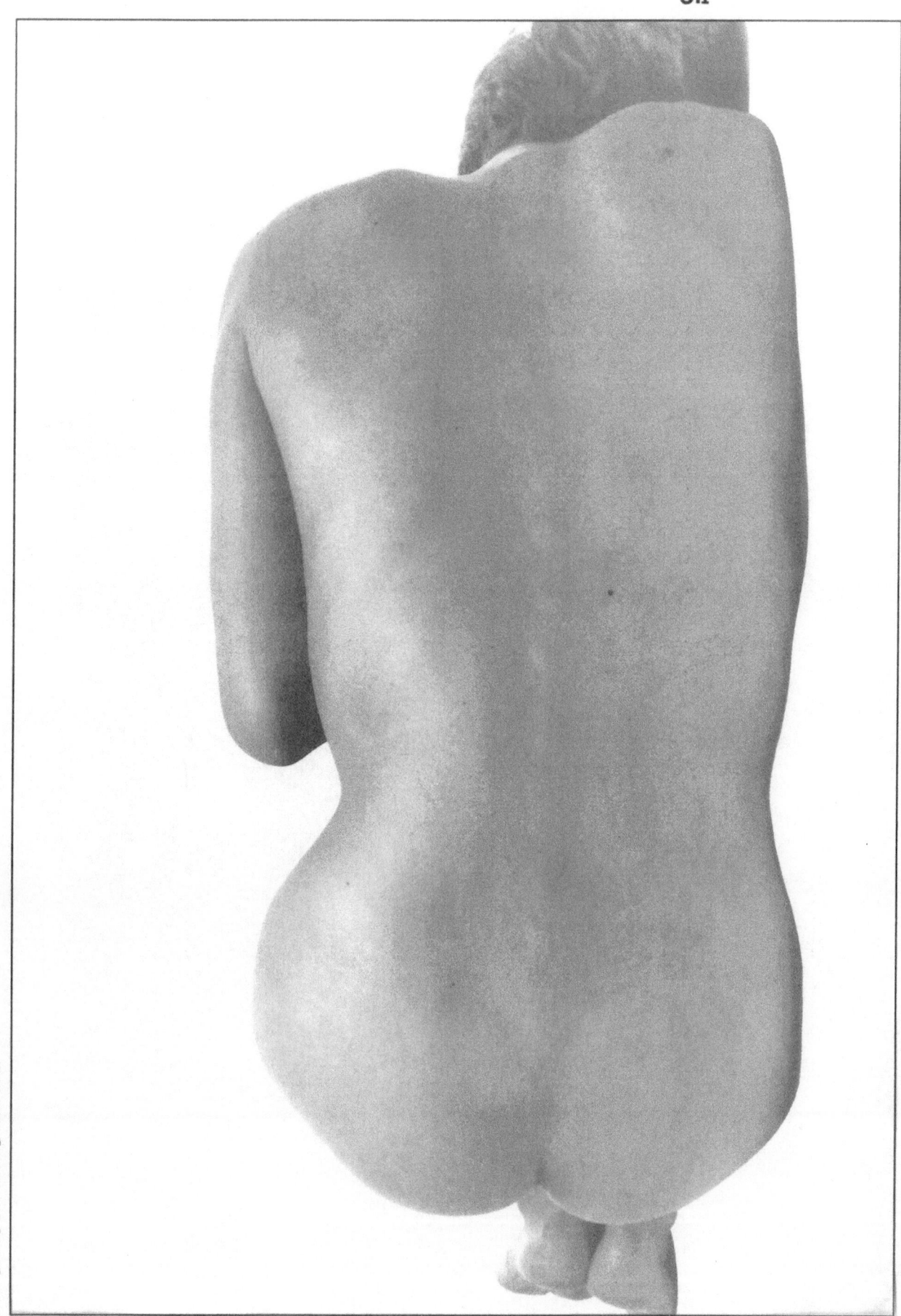

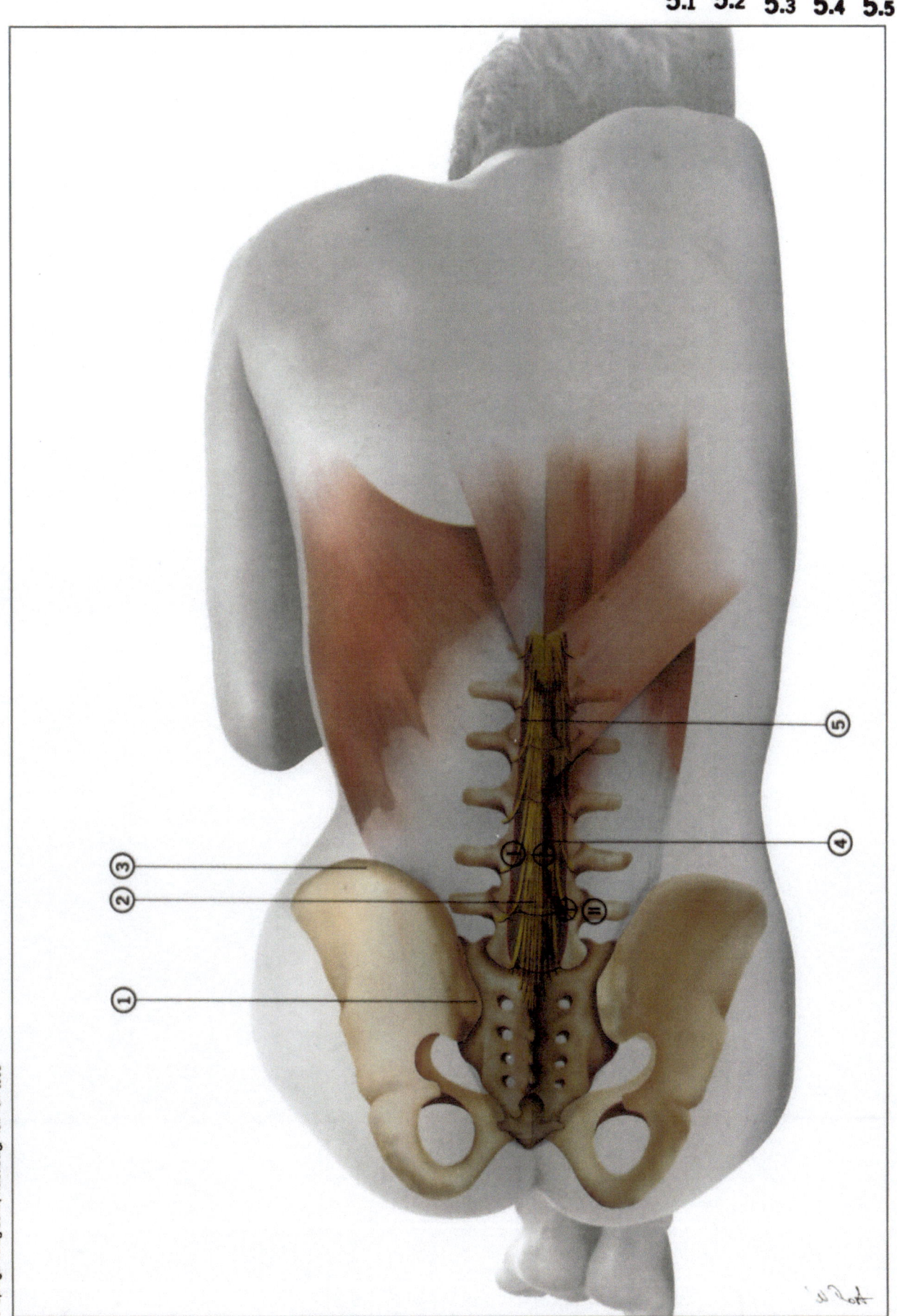

① Injection site for midline approach to L3–4 interspace. ⑪ Injection site for paramedian approach to L3–4 interspace. ① Posterior superior iliac spine. ② Spinous process of L4. ③ Superior iliac crest. ④ Spinous process of L3. ⑤ Lamina of L1

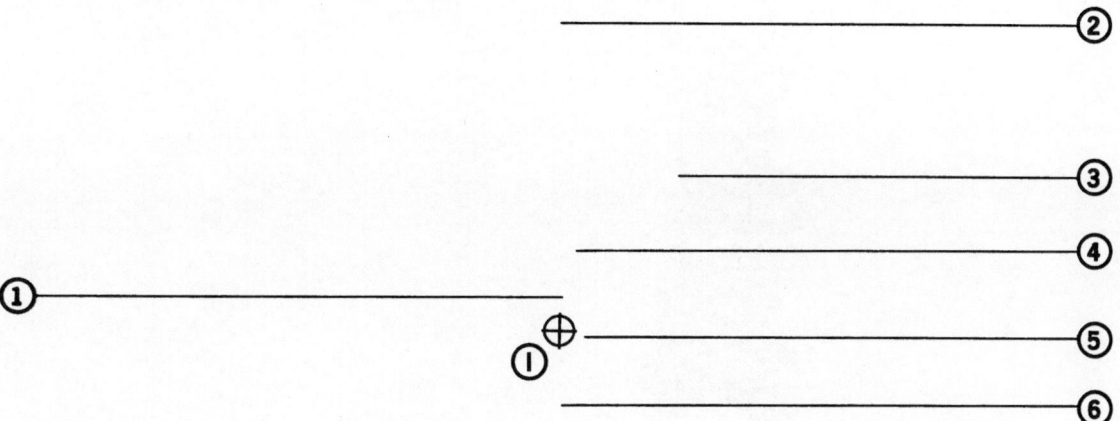

⊕ Injection site for caudal approach. ① Sacral hiatus. ② Spinous process of L5. ③ Posterior superior iliac spine. ④ Articular ridge. ⑤ Sacral cornu.
⑥ Coccyx

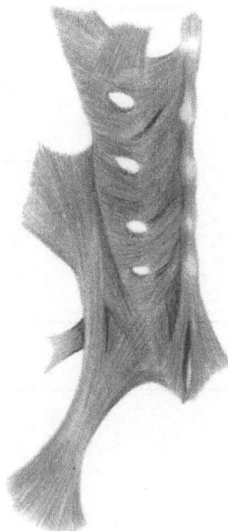

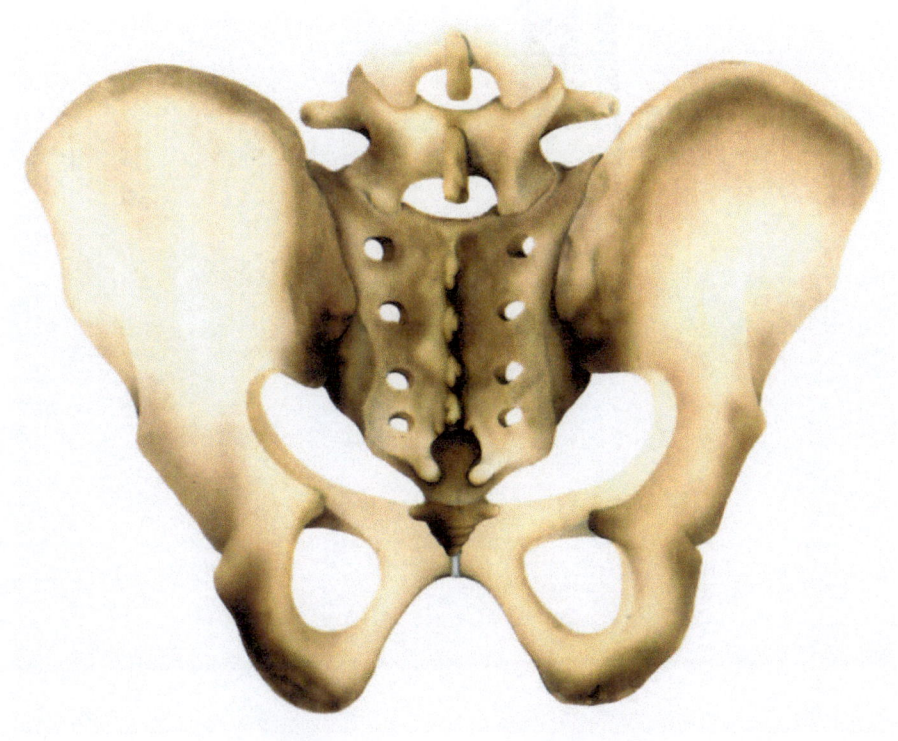

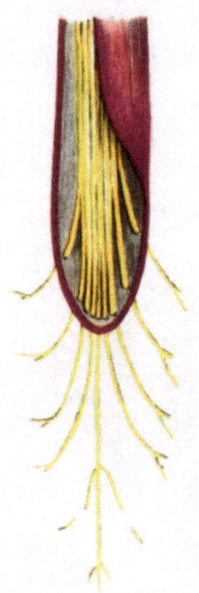

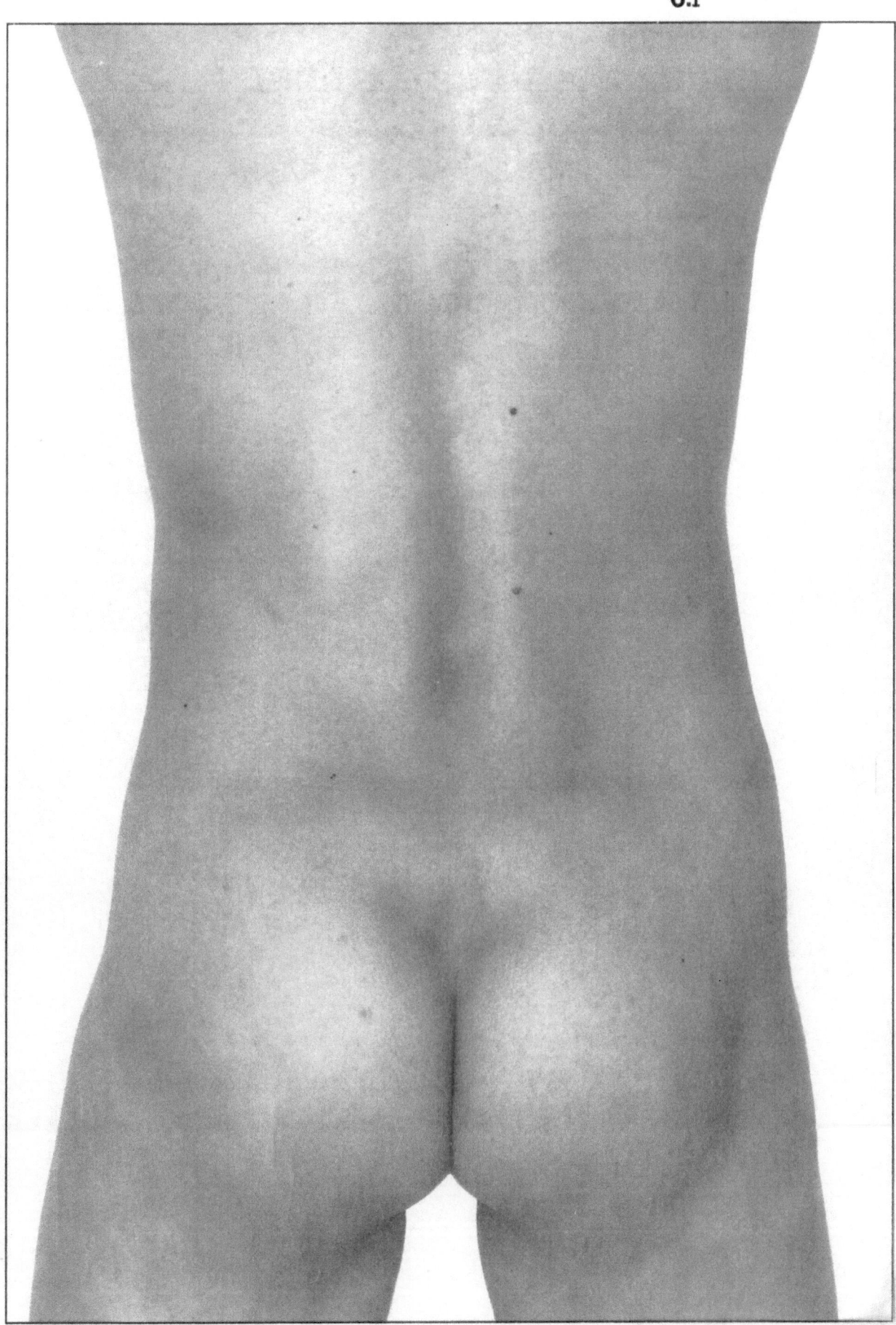

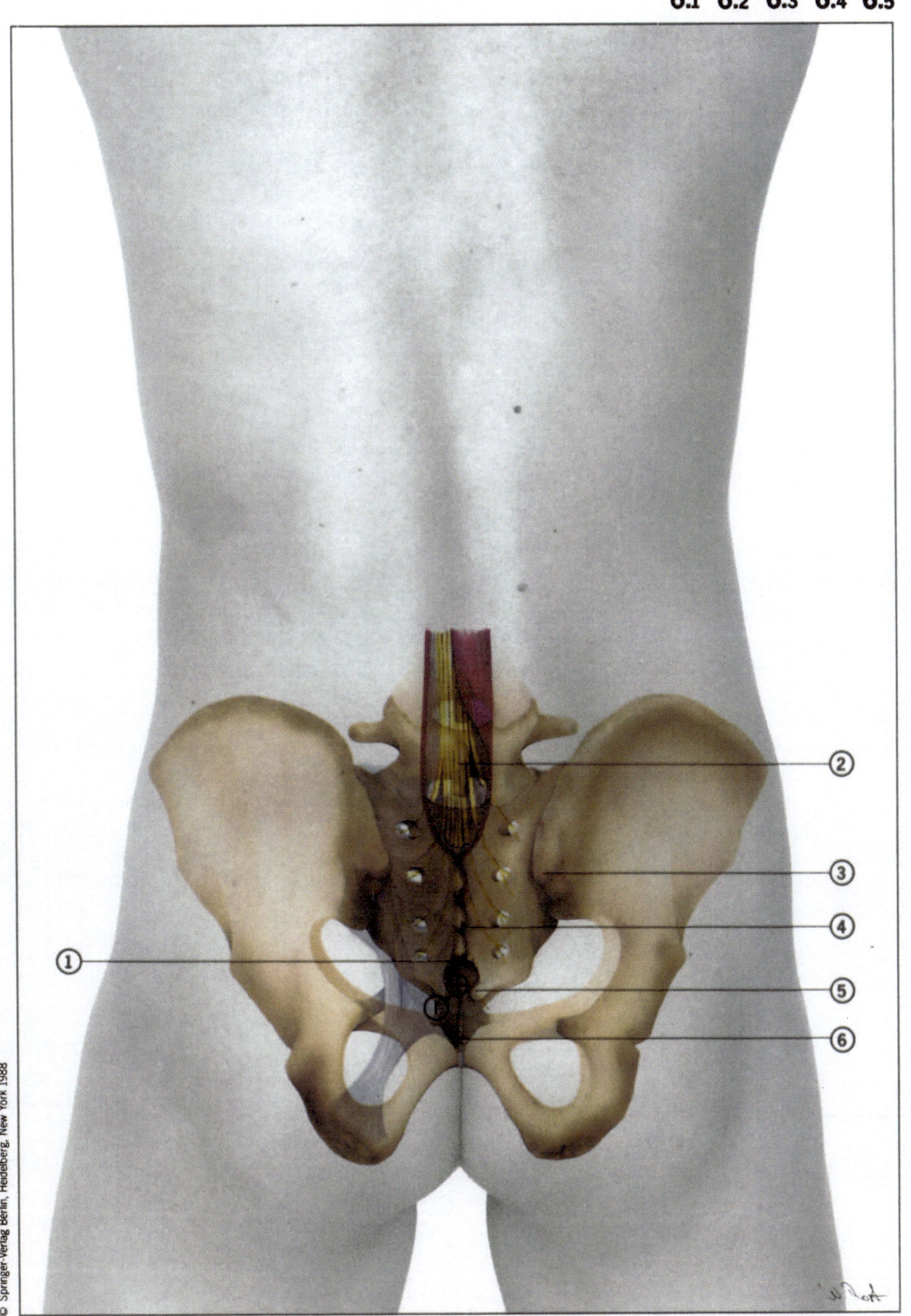

① Injection site for caudal approach. ① Sacral hiatus. ② Spinous process of L5. ③ Posterior superior iliac spine. ④ Articular ridge. ⑤ Sacral cornu. ⑥ Coccyx

① Injection site for interscalene approach. ① Sternocleidomastoid muscle. ② Trapezius muscle. ③ Scalenus medius muscle. ④ Clavicle.
⑤ Scalenus anterior muscle. ⑥ Cricoid cartilage. ⑦ Brachial plexus. ⑧ Clavicular head of sternocleidomastoid muscle. ⑨ Sternal head of sternocleidomastoid muscle
Note: For clarity of presentation, the cervical portion of the spine is not shown rotated to correspond to the rotation of the neck. This does not affect the landmarks for blocks in the neck

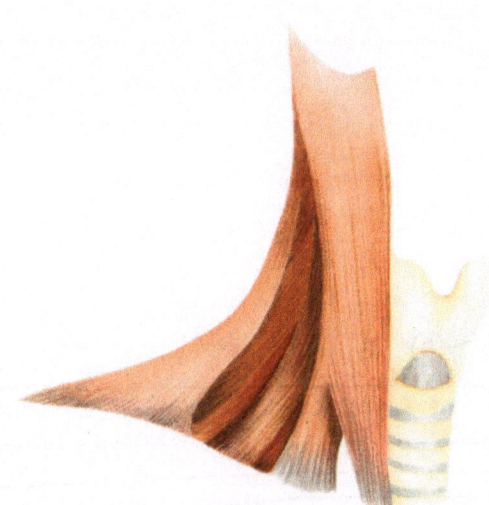

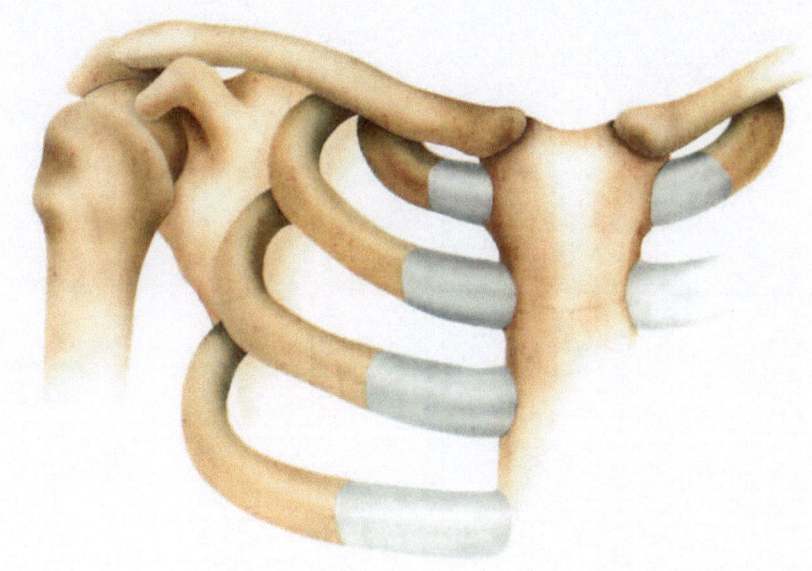

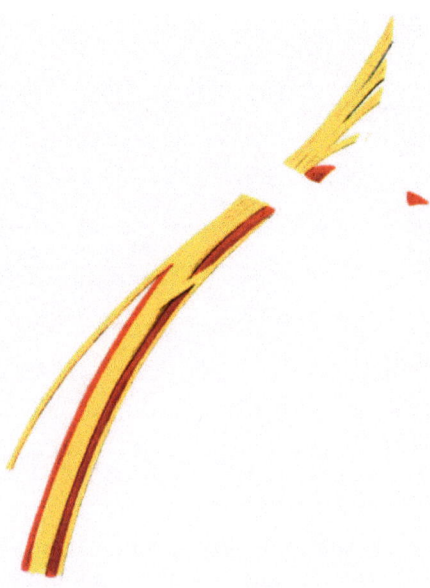

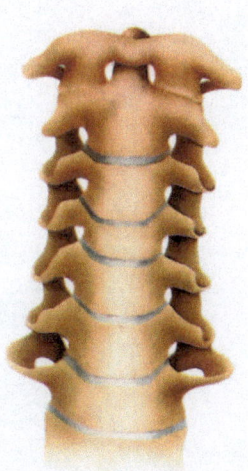

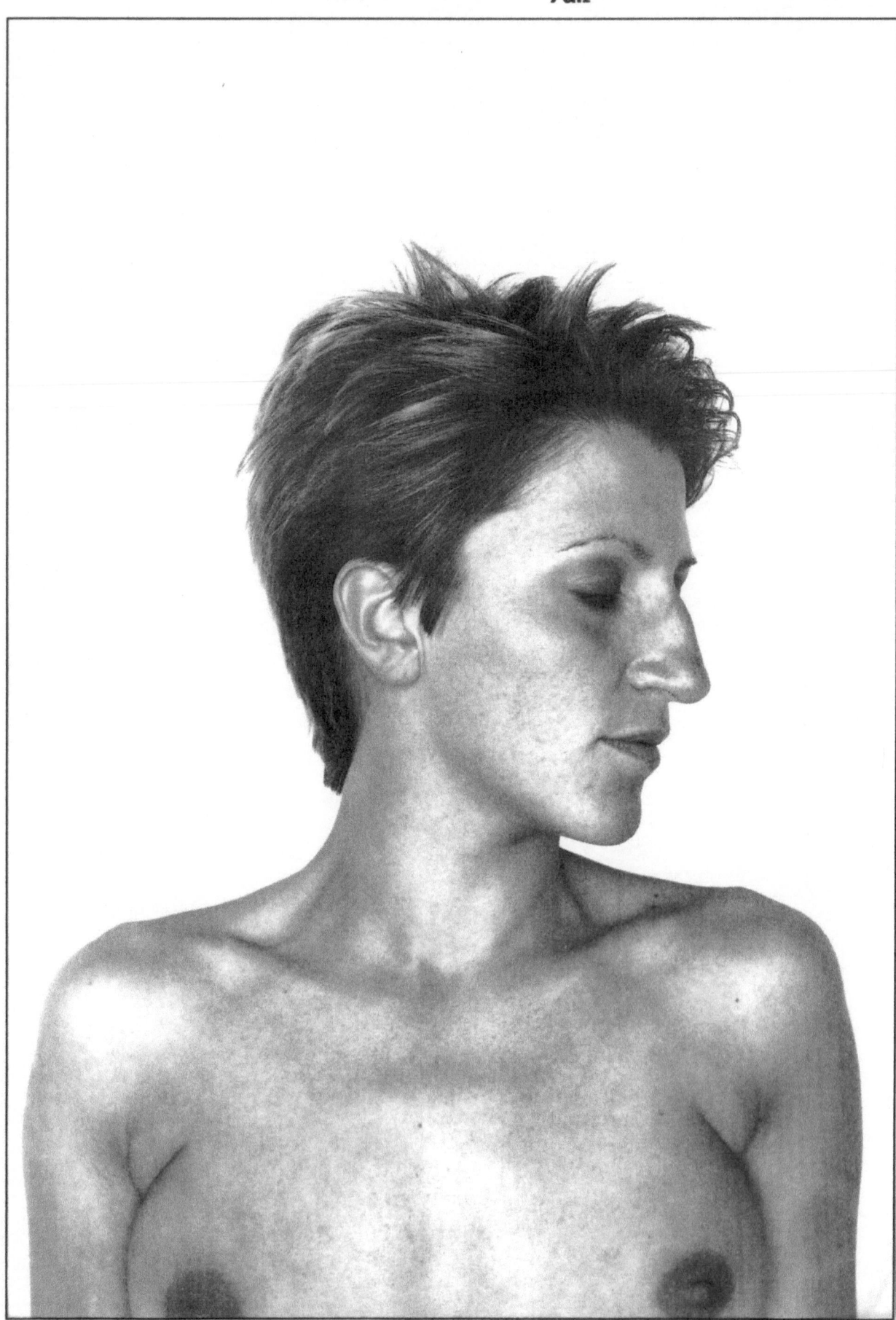

7a

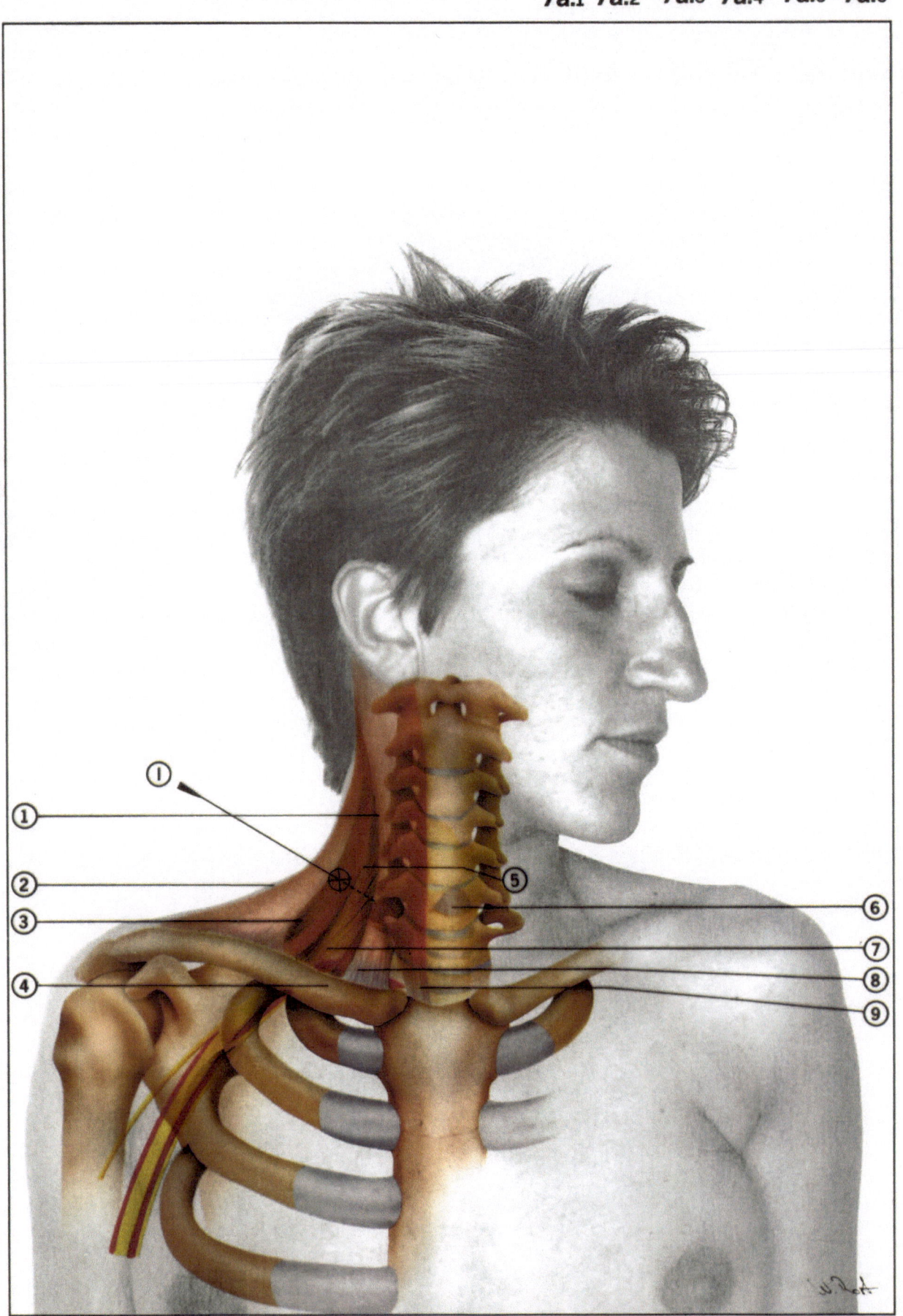

① Injection site for interscalene approach. ① Sternocleidomastoid muscle. ② Trapezius muscle. ③ Scalenus medius muscle. ④ Clavicle. ⑤ Scalenus anterior muscle. ⑥ Cricoid cartilage. ⑦ Brachial plexus. ⑧ Clavicular head of sternocleidomastoid muscle. ⑨ Sternal head of sternocleidomastoid muscle

Note: For clarity of presentation, the cervical portion of the spine is not shown rotated to correspond to the rotation of the neck. This does not affect the landmarks for blocks in the neck

Ⓘ Injection site for supraclavicular block. Ⓤ Injection site for subclavian perivascular block. ① Sternocleidomastoid muscle. ② Trapezius muscle. ③ Scalenus medius muscle. ④ Clavicle. ⑤ Scalenus anterior muscle. ⑥ Cricoid cartilage. ⑦ Brachial plexus. ⑧ Clavicular head of sternocleidomastoid muscle. ⑨ Sternal head of sternocleidomastoid muscle

Note: For clarity of presentation, the cervical portion of the spine is not shown rotated to correspond to the rotation of the neck. This does not affect the landmarks for blocks in the neck

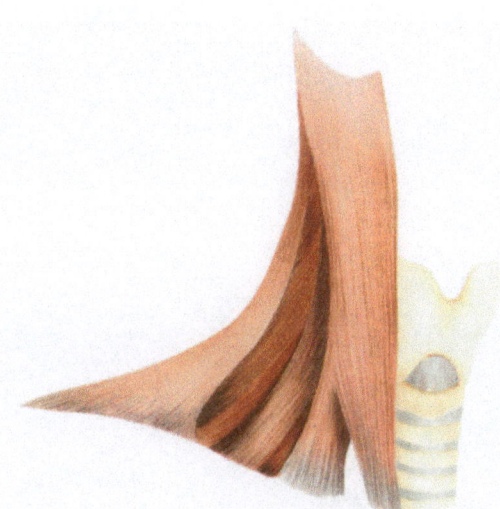

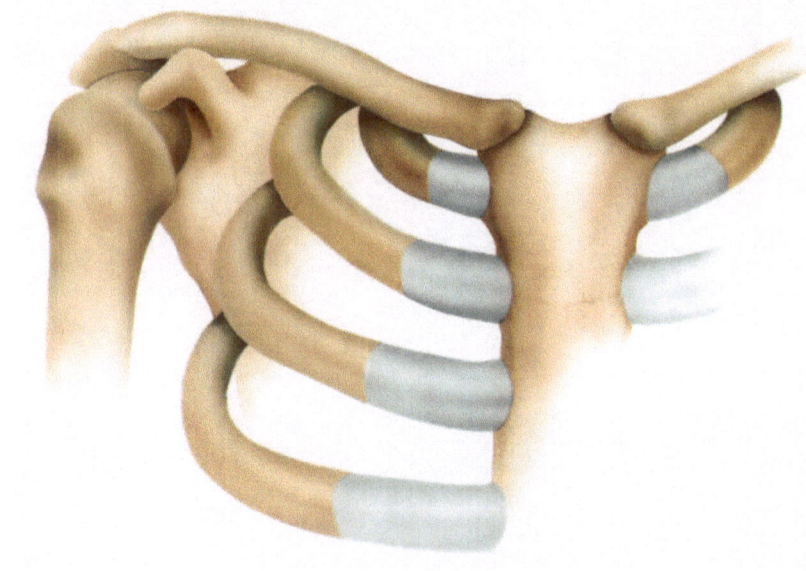

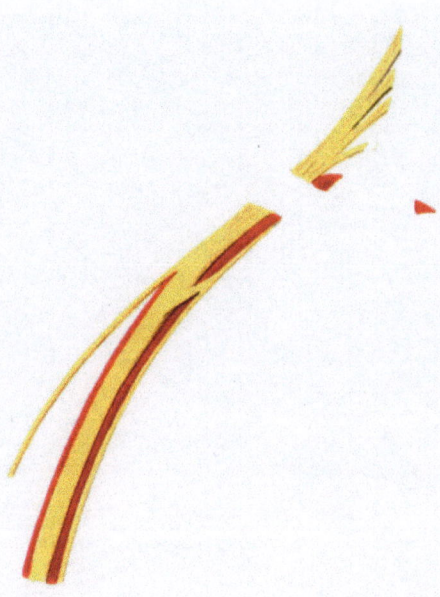

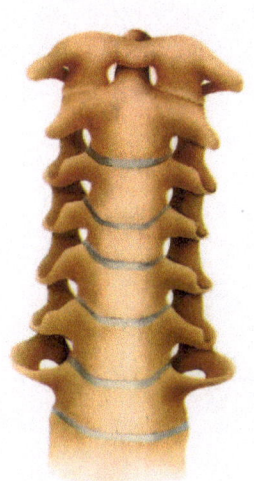

7b.1

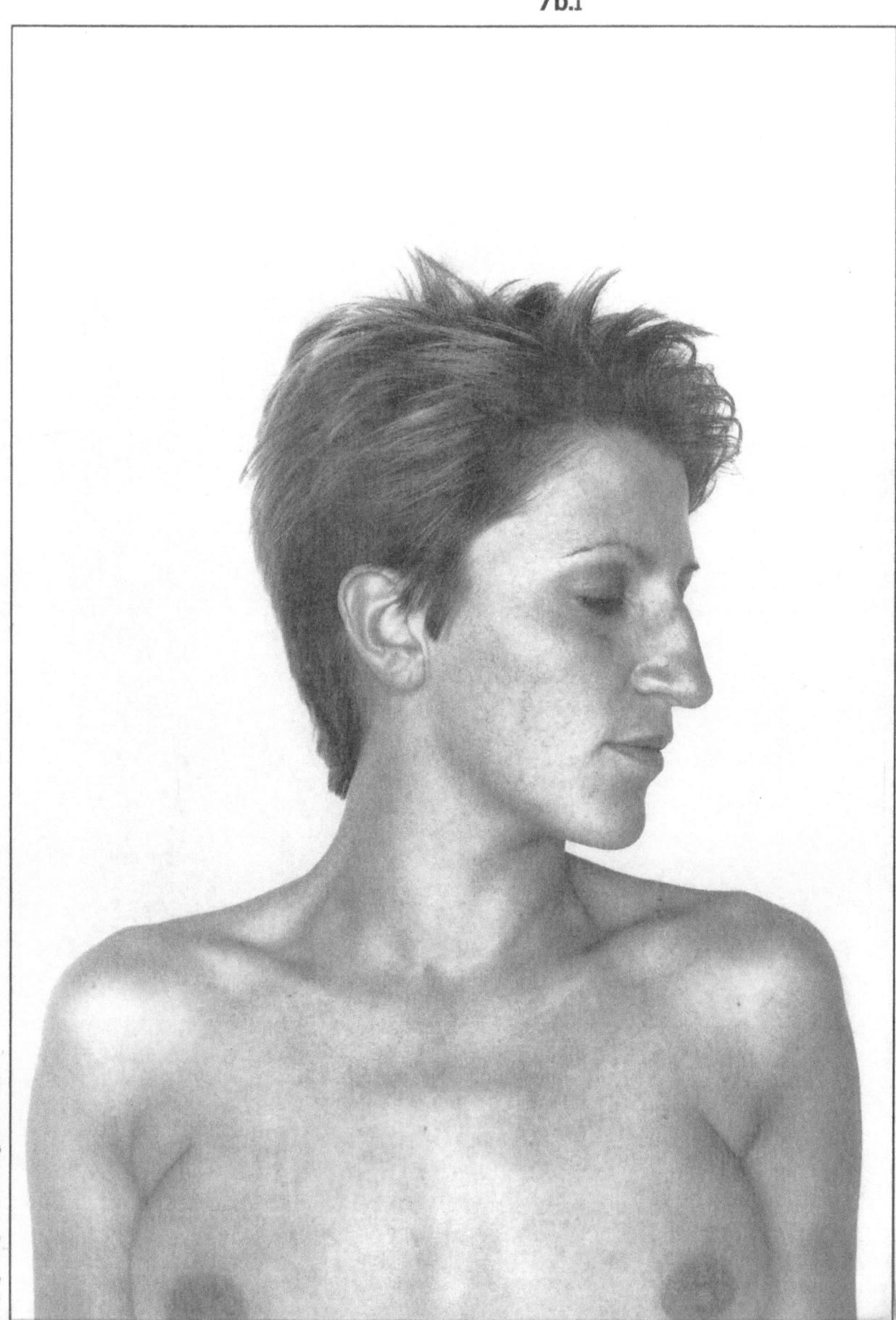

7b

Brachial Plexus Block: Supraclavicular Approach

Brachial Plexus Block: Supraclavicular Approach

7b

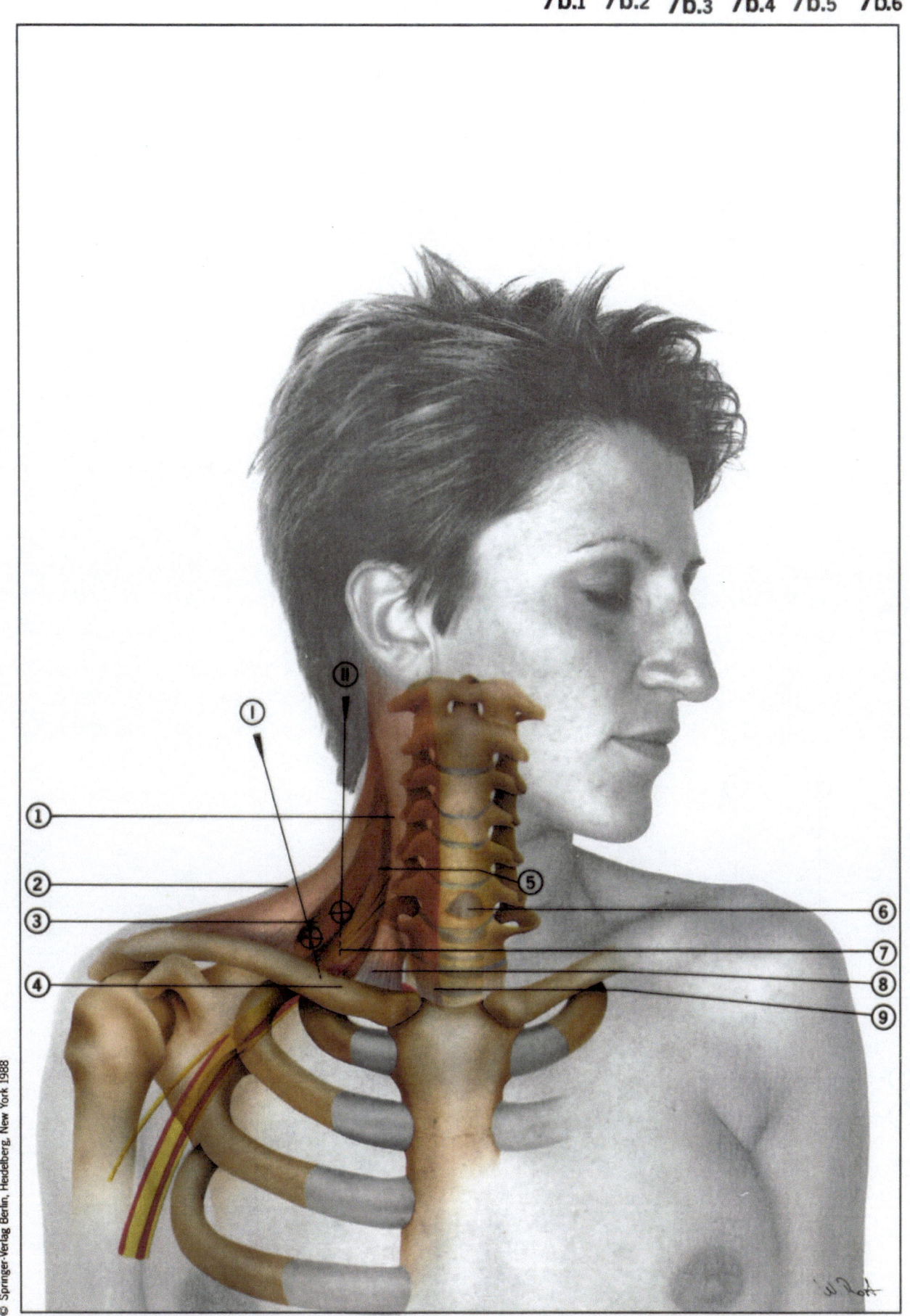

① Injection site for supraclavicular block. ⑪ Injection site for subclavian perivascular block. ① Sternocleidomastoid muscle. ② Trapezius muscle.
③ Scalenus medius muscle. ④ Clavicle. ⑤ Scalenus anterior muscle. ⑥ Cricoid cartilage. ⑦ Brachial plexus. ⑧ Clavicular head of
sternocleidomastoid muscle. ⑨ Sternal head of sternocleidomastoid muscle
Note: For clarity of presentation, the cervical portion of the spine is not shown rotated to correspond to the rotation of the neck. This does not
affect the landmarks for blocks in the neck

③ ② ①

④

⑤

⑥

① Injection site for infraclavicular approach. ① Midpoint of clavicle. ② Cords of the brachial plexus. ③ Axillary artery. ④ Axillary vein. ⑤ Rib cage.
⑥ Anterior chest wall
Note: For clarity of presentation, the cervical portion of the spine is not shown rotated to correspond to the rotation of the neck. This does not affect the landmarks for blocks in the neck

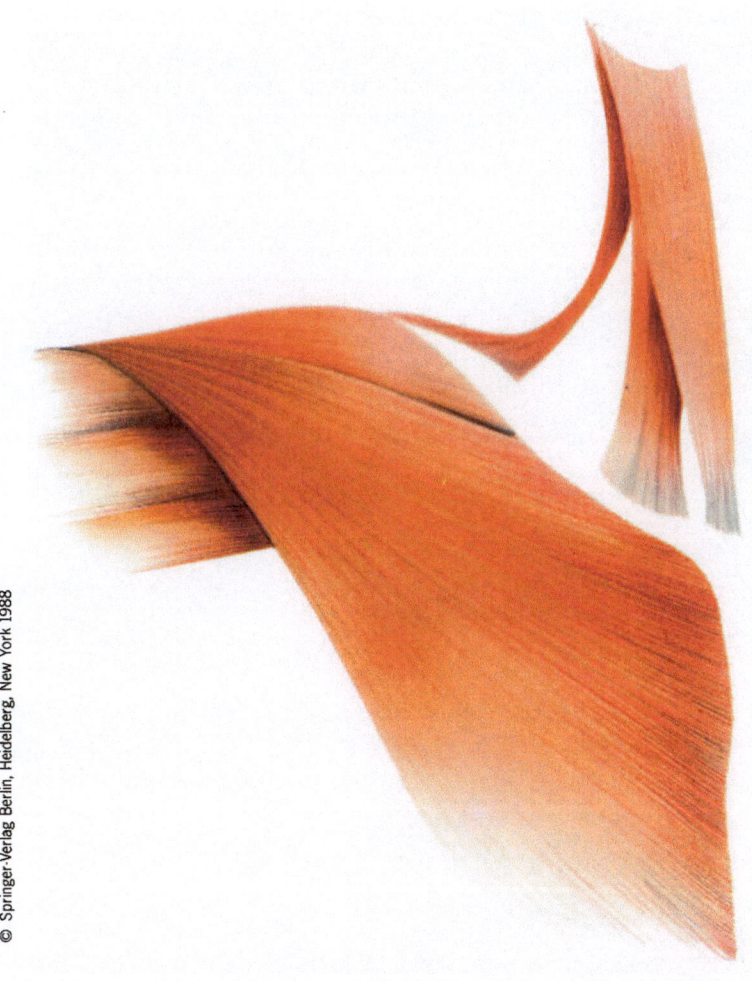

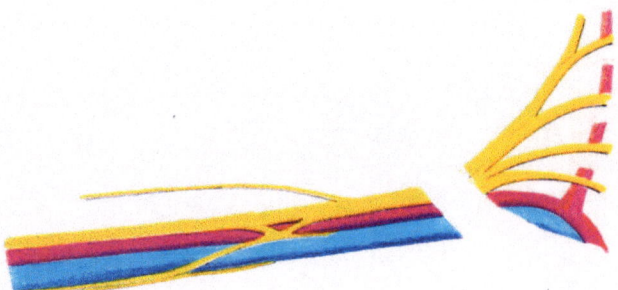

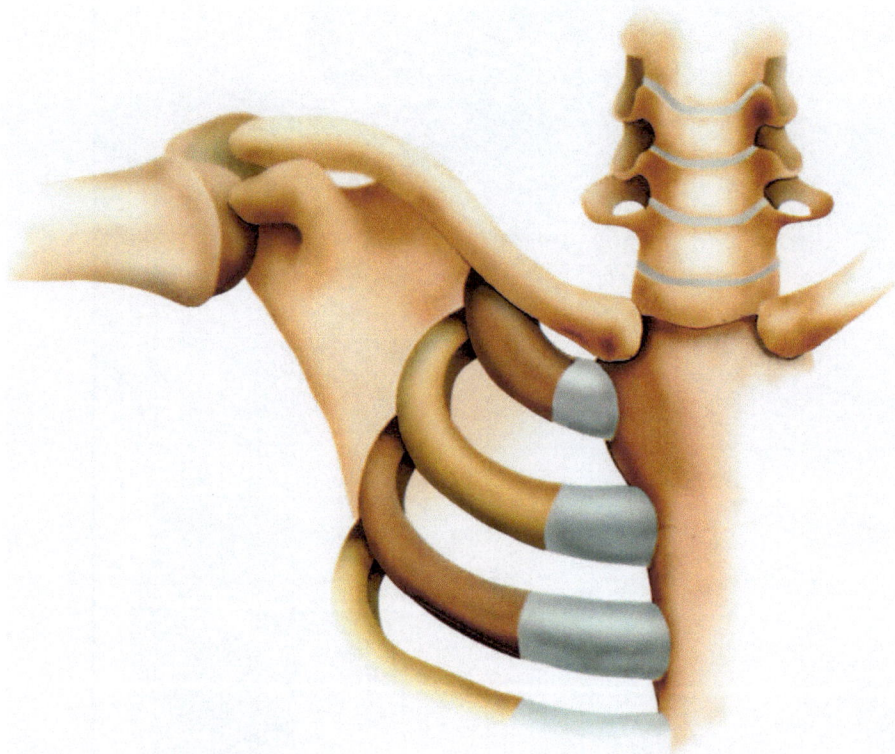

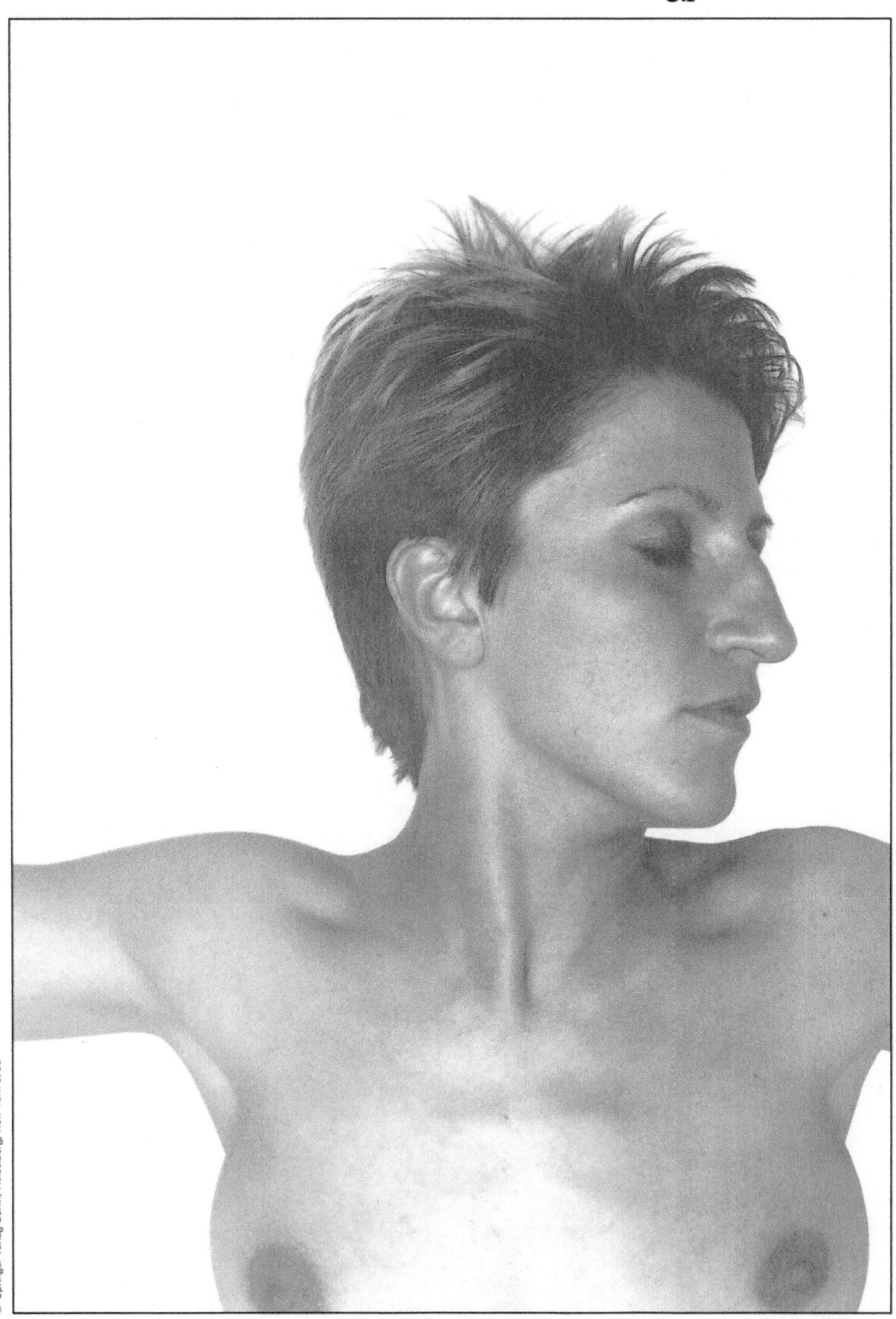

Brachial Plexus Block: Infraclavicular Approach

8

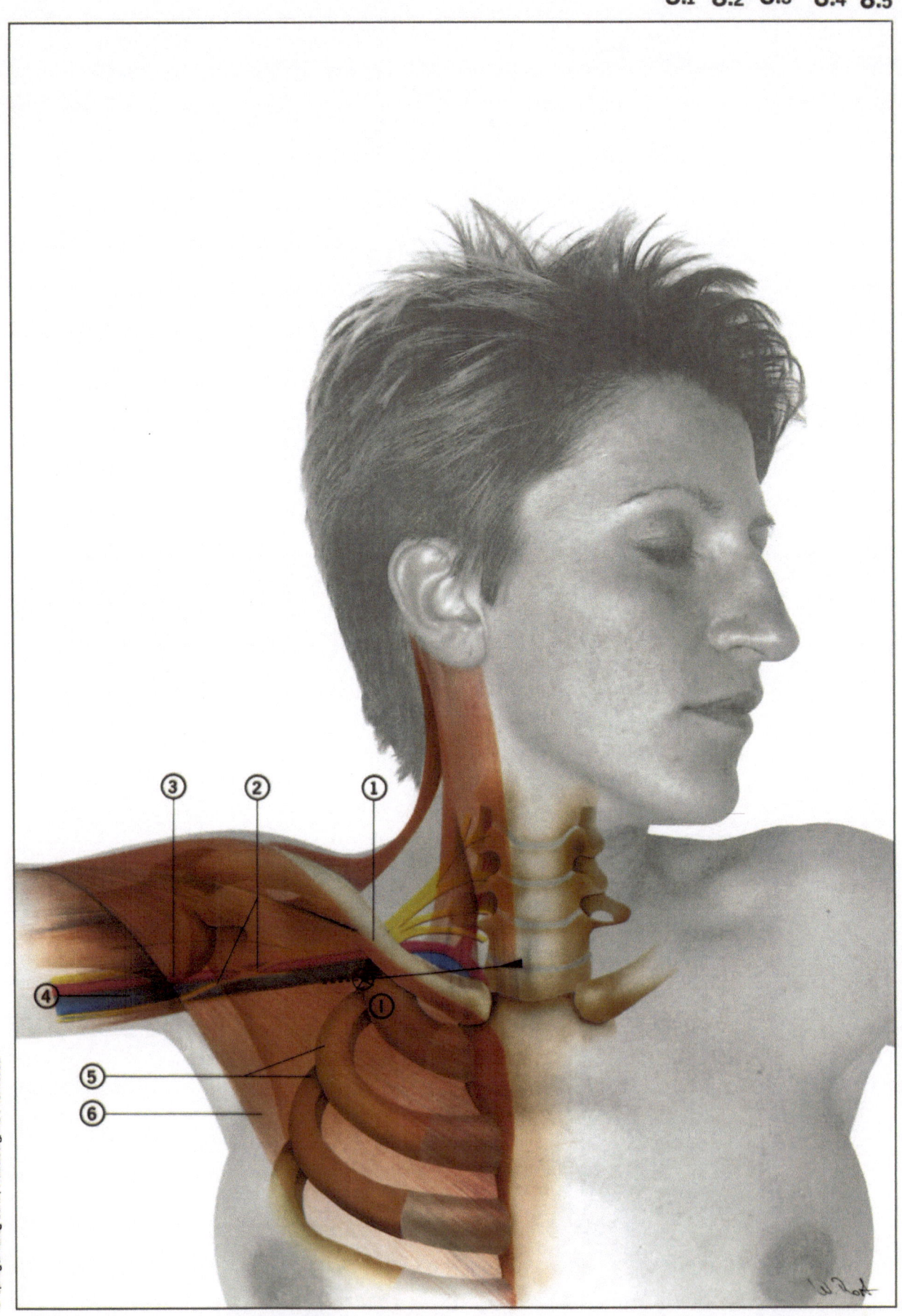

① Injection site for infraclavicular approach. ① Midpoint of clavicle. ② Cords of the brachial plexus. ③ Axillary artery. ④ Axillary vein. ⑤ Rib cage. ⑥ Anterior chest wall

Note: For clarity of presentation, the cervical portion of the spine is not shown rotated to correspond to the rotation of the neck. This does not affect the landmarks for blocks in the neck

① Injection site for axillary approach. ① Humerus. ② Biceps muscle. ③ Brachial plexus with axillary vessels. ④ Head of humerus. ⑤ Anterior chest wall (pectoralis major muscle). ⑥ Posterior chest wall (latissimus dorsi and teres major muscles). ⑦ Triceps muscle

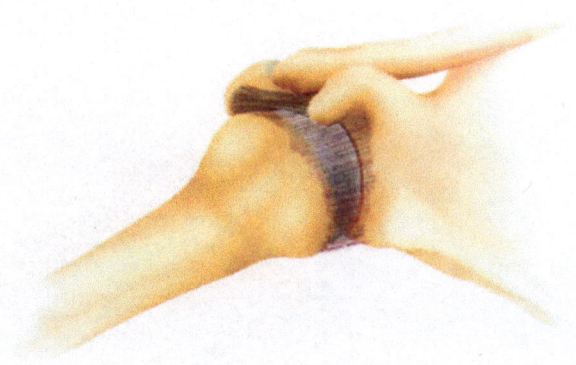

© Springer-Verlag Berlin, Heidelberg, New York 1988

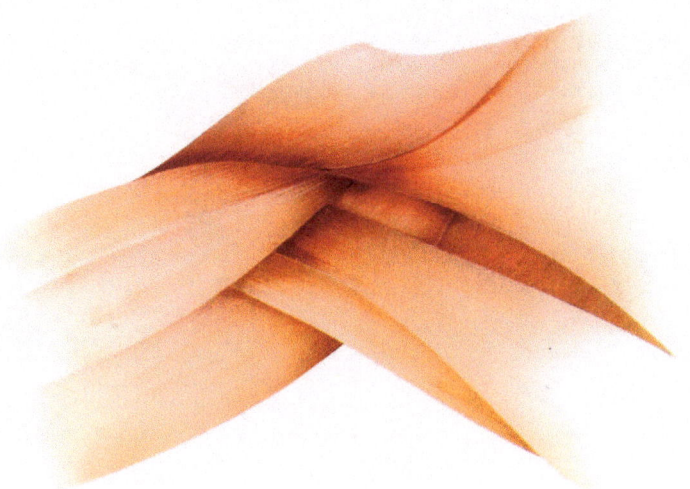

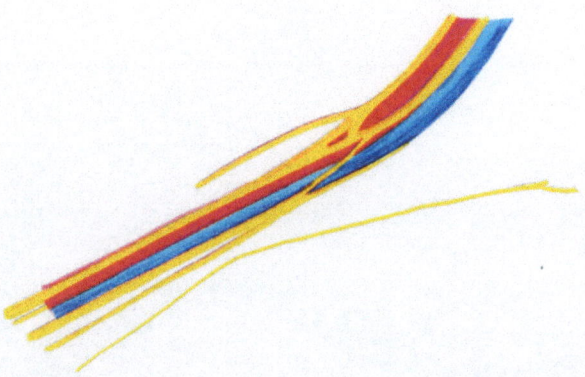

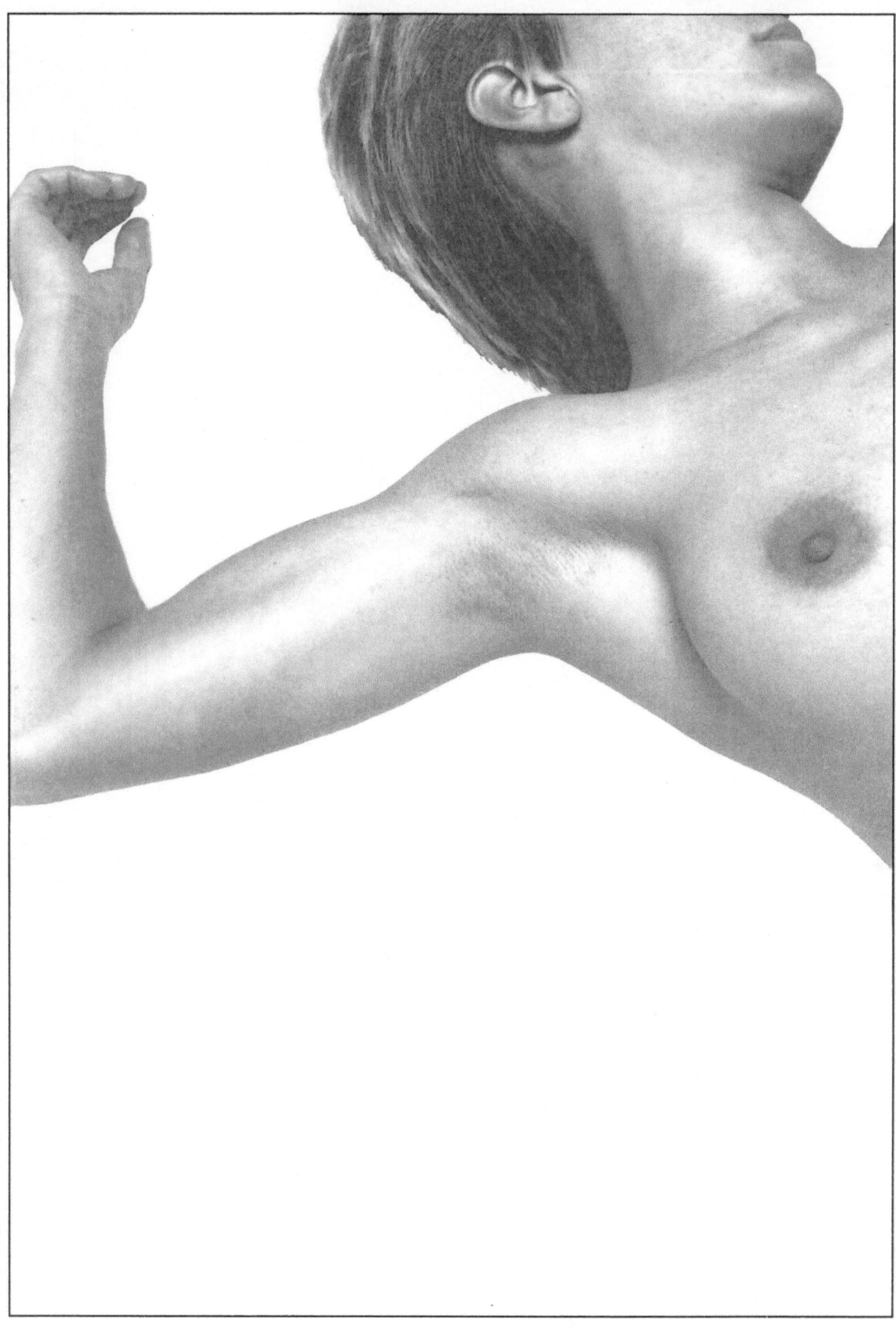

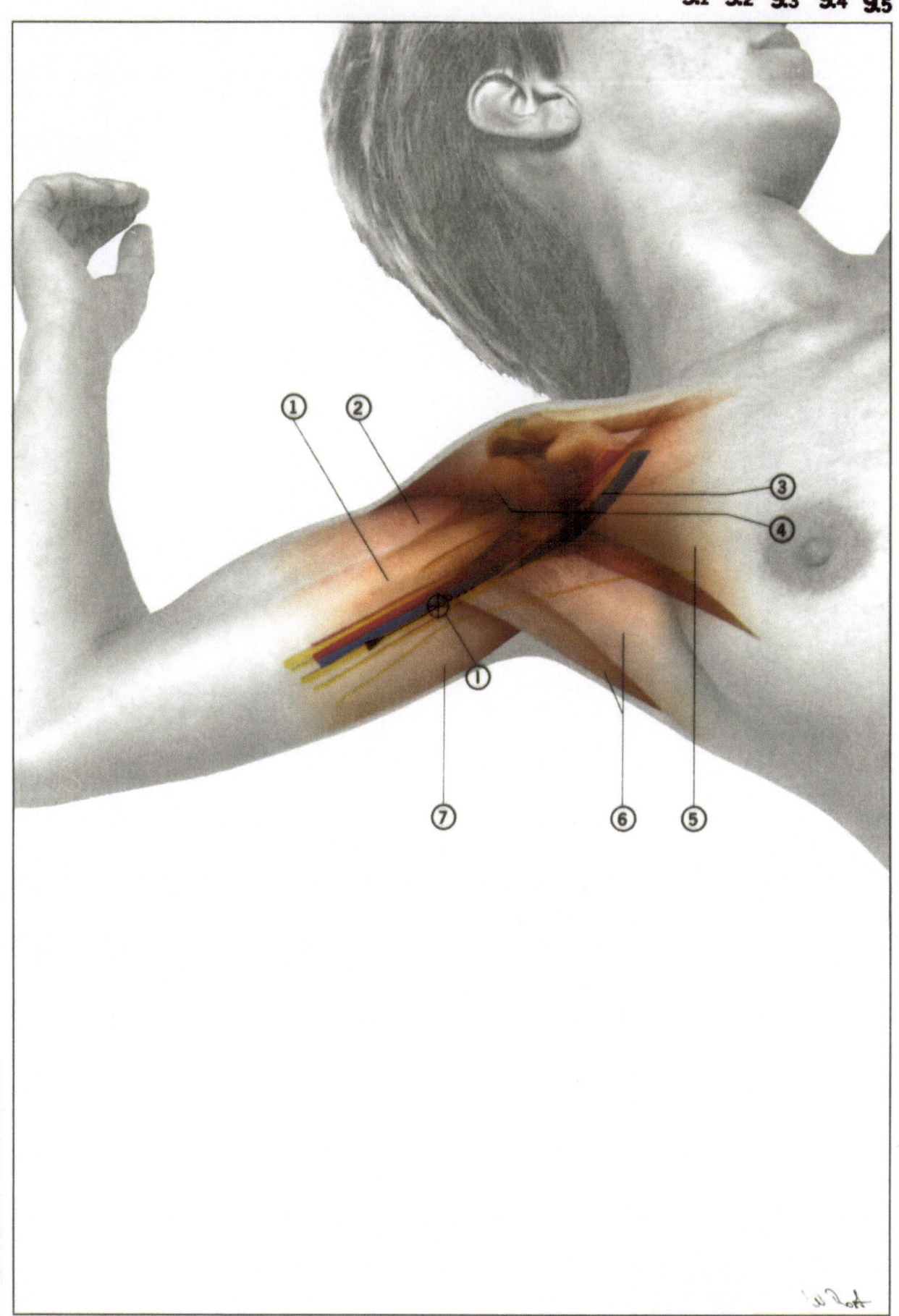

⊕ Injection site for axillary approach. ① Humerus. ② Biceps muscle. ③ Brachial plexus with axillary vessels. ④ Head of humerus. ⑤ Anterior chest wall (pectoralis major muscle). ⑥ Posterior chest wall (latissimus dorsi and teres major muscles). ⑦ Triceps muscle

① Injection site for suprascapular nerve block at scapular notch. A – – – –A: Line demarcating scapular spine. B – – – –B: Line intersecting midpoint of scapular spine. C: Midpoint of scapular spine. ① Scapular nerve at scapular notch. ② Scapular spine. ③ Infraspinatus muscle. ④ Scapular angle. ⑤ Supraspinatus muscle

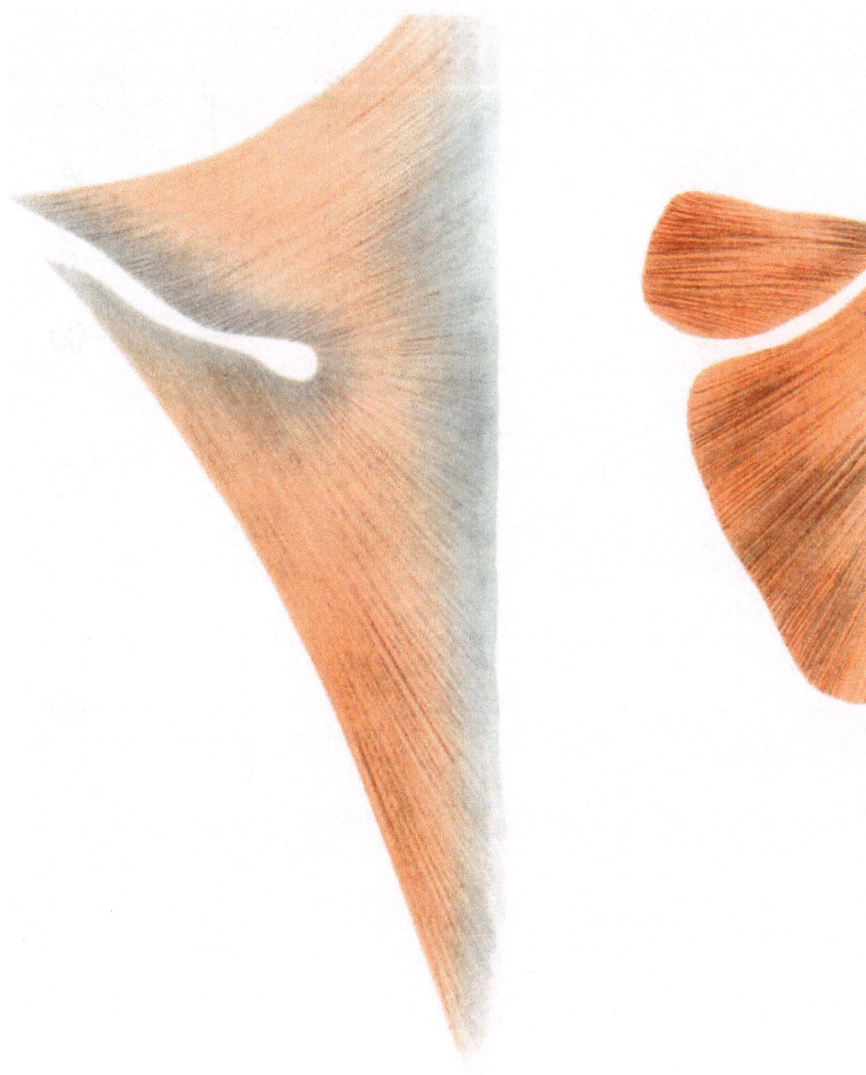

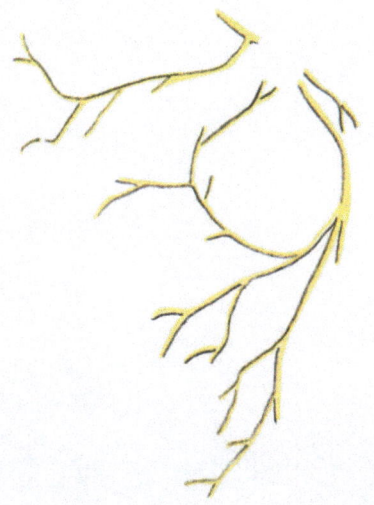

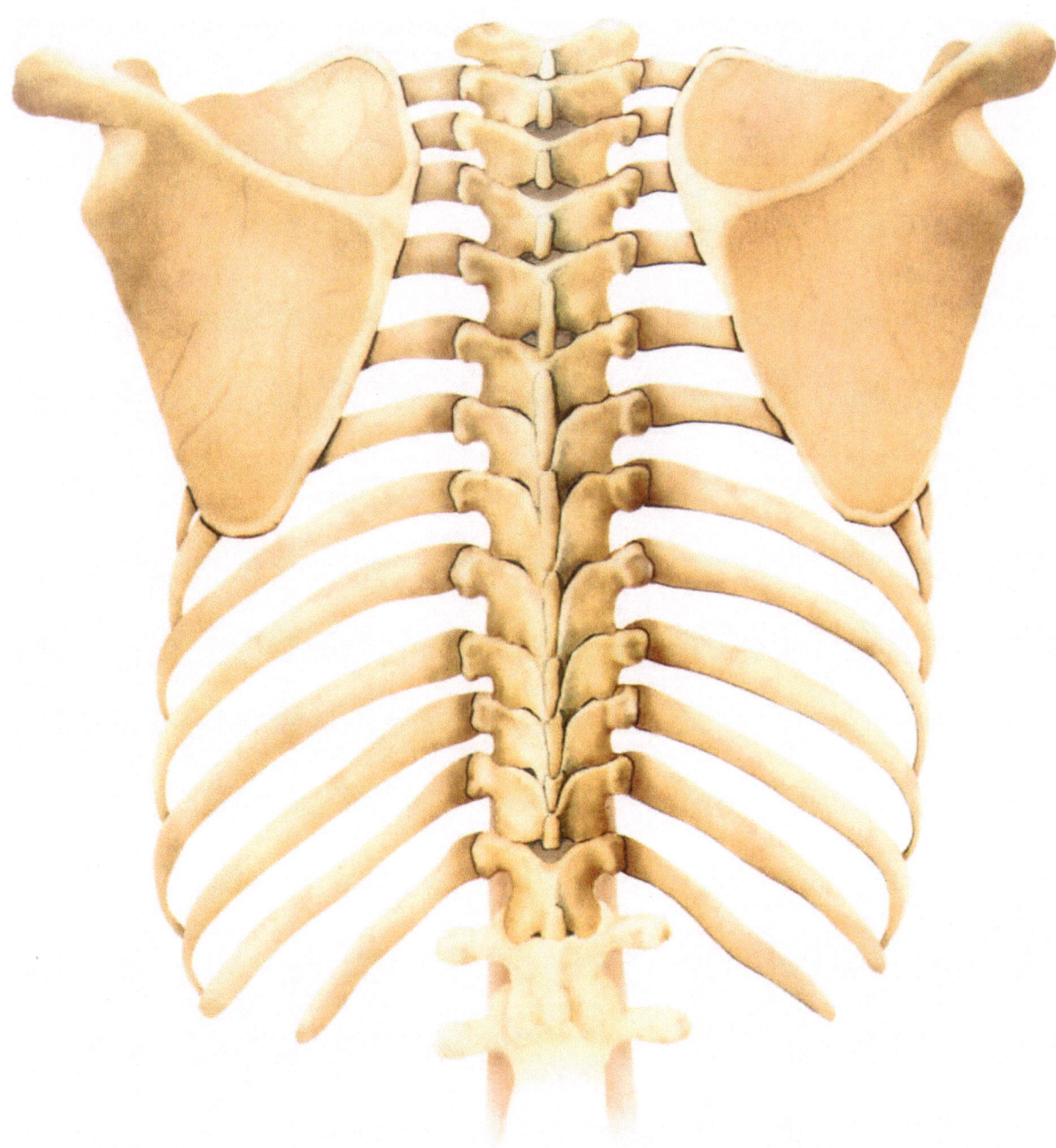

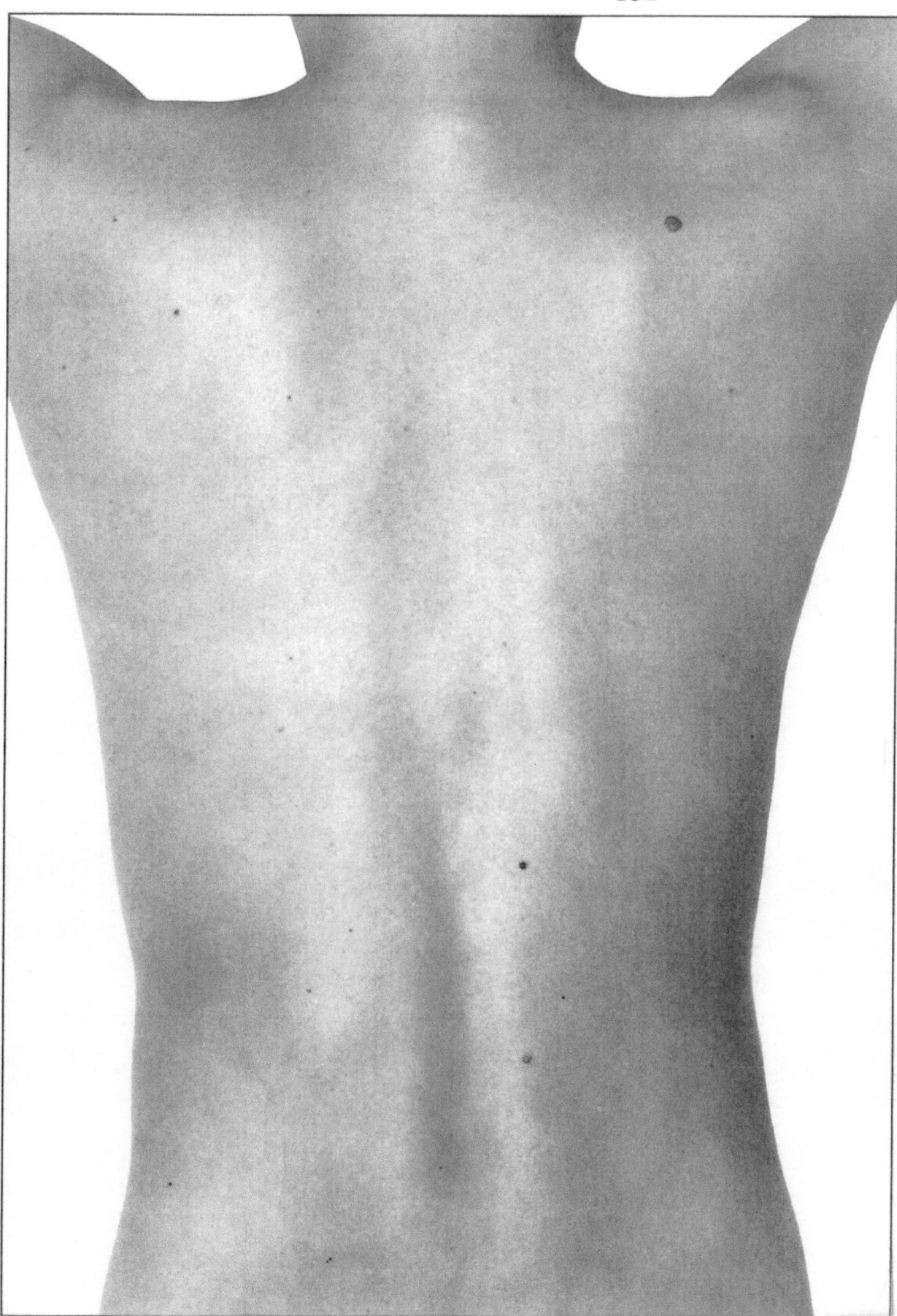

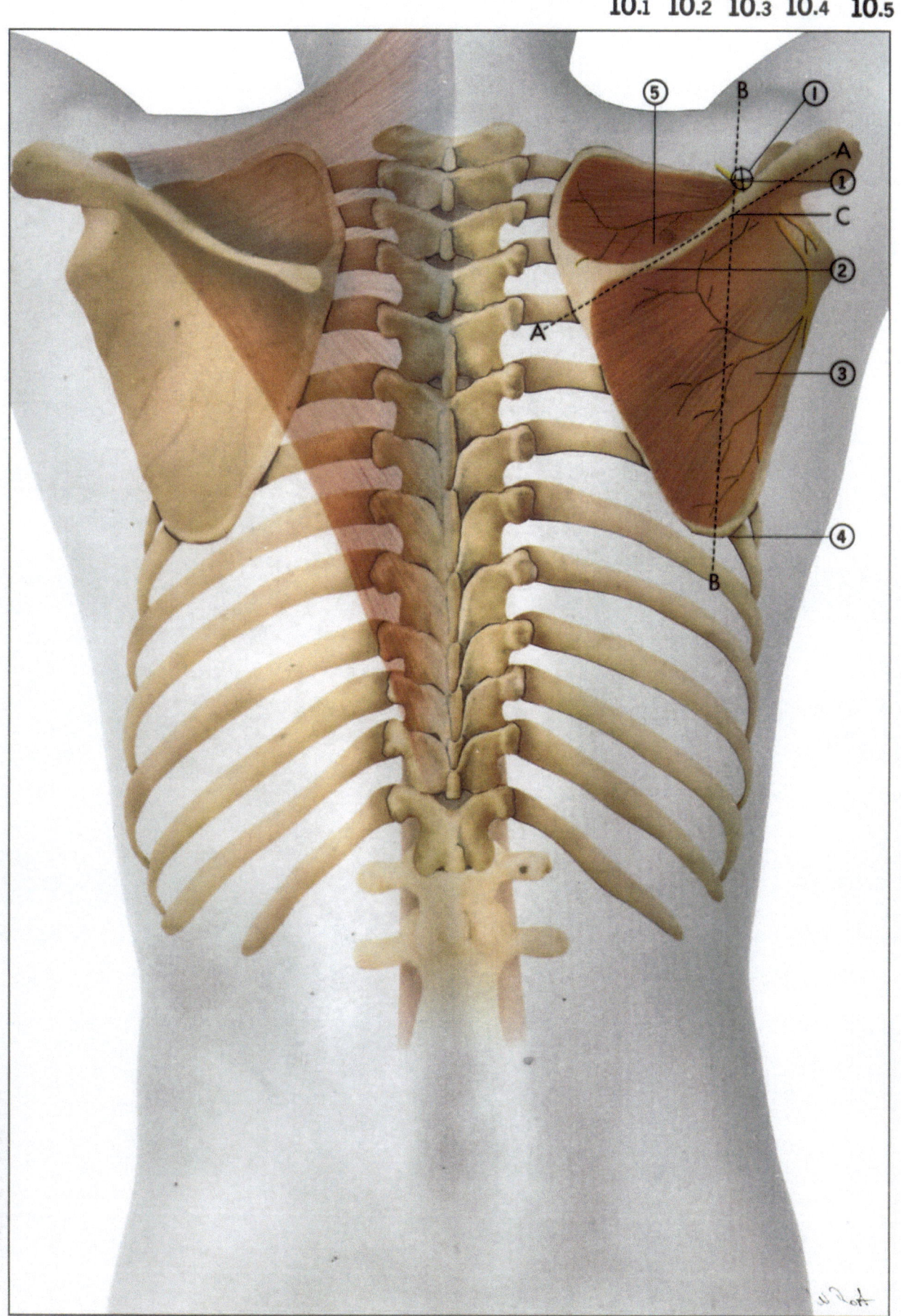

10

① Injection site for suprascapular nerve block at scapular notch. A – – – –A: Line demarcating scapular spine. B – – – –B: Line intersecting midpoint of scapular spine. C: Midpoint of scapular spine. ① Scapular nerve at scapular notch. ② Scapular spine. ③ Infraspinatus muscle. ④ Scapular angle. ⑤ Supraspinatus muscle

①

④

⑤

②

⑥

⑦

Ⓘ Ⓘ Ⓘ

⑧

③

Ⓘ Injection site for radial and musculocutaneous nerve block. Ⓘ Injection site for median nerve block at elbow. ① Biceps muscle.
② Musculocutaneous nerve. ③ Radial nerve. ④ Brachial artery. ⑤ Ulnar nerve. ⑥ Tendon of biceps muscle. ⑦ Crease at the cubital fossa. ⑧ Ulna

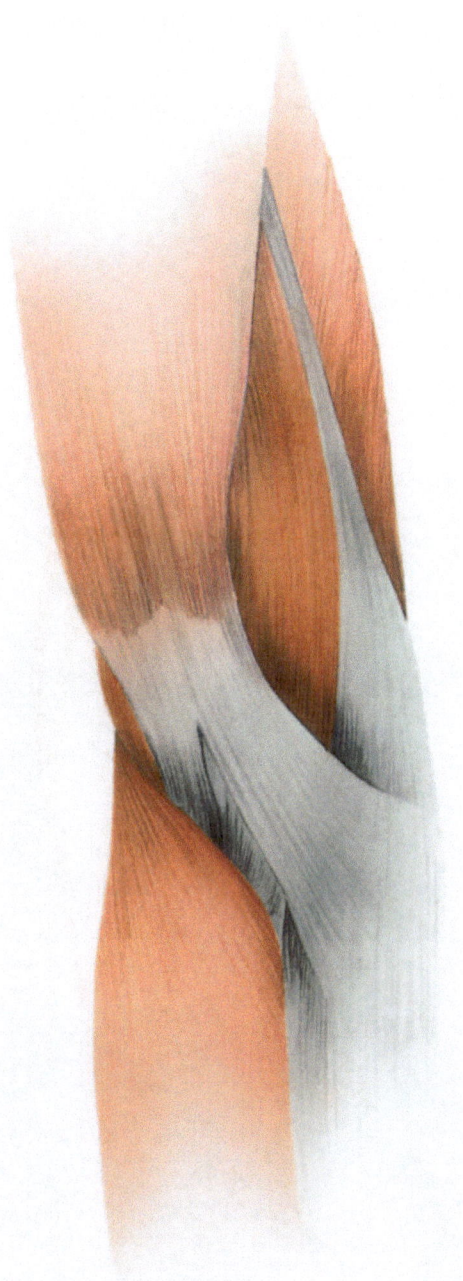

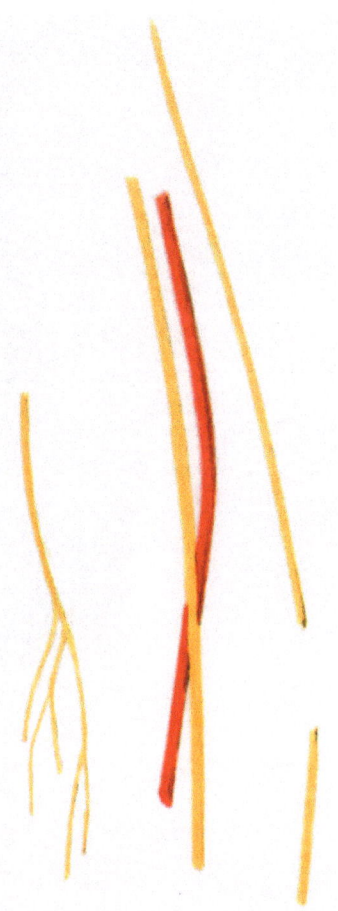

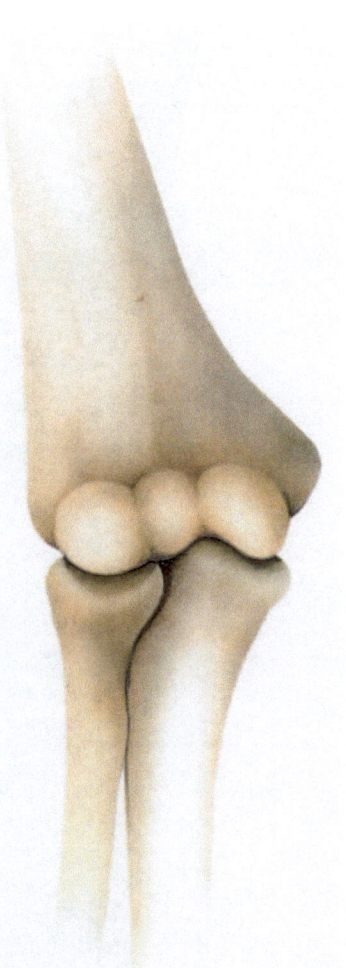

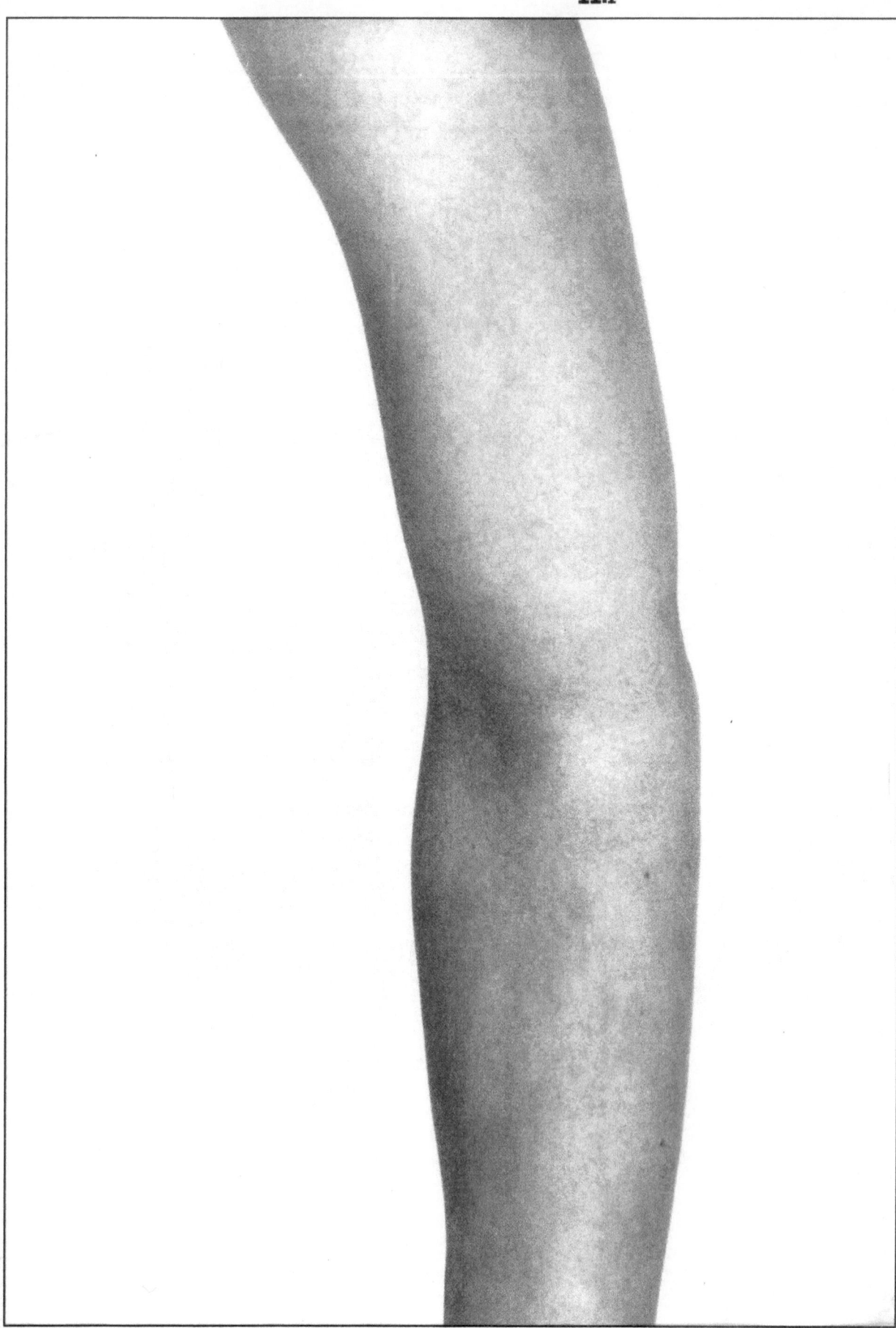

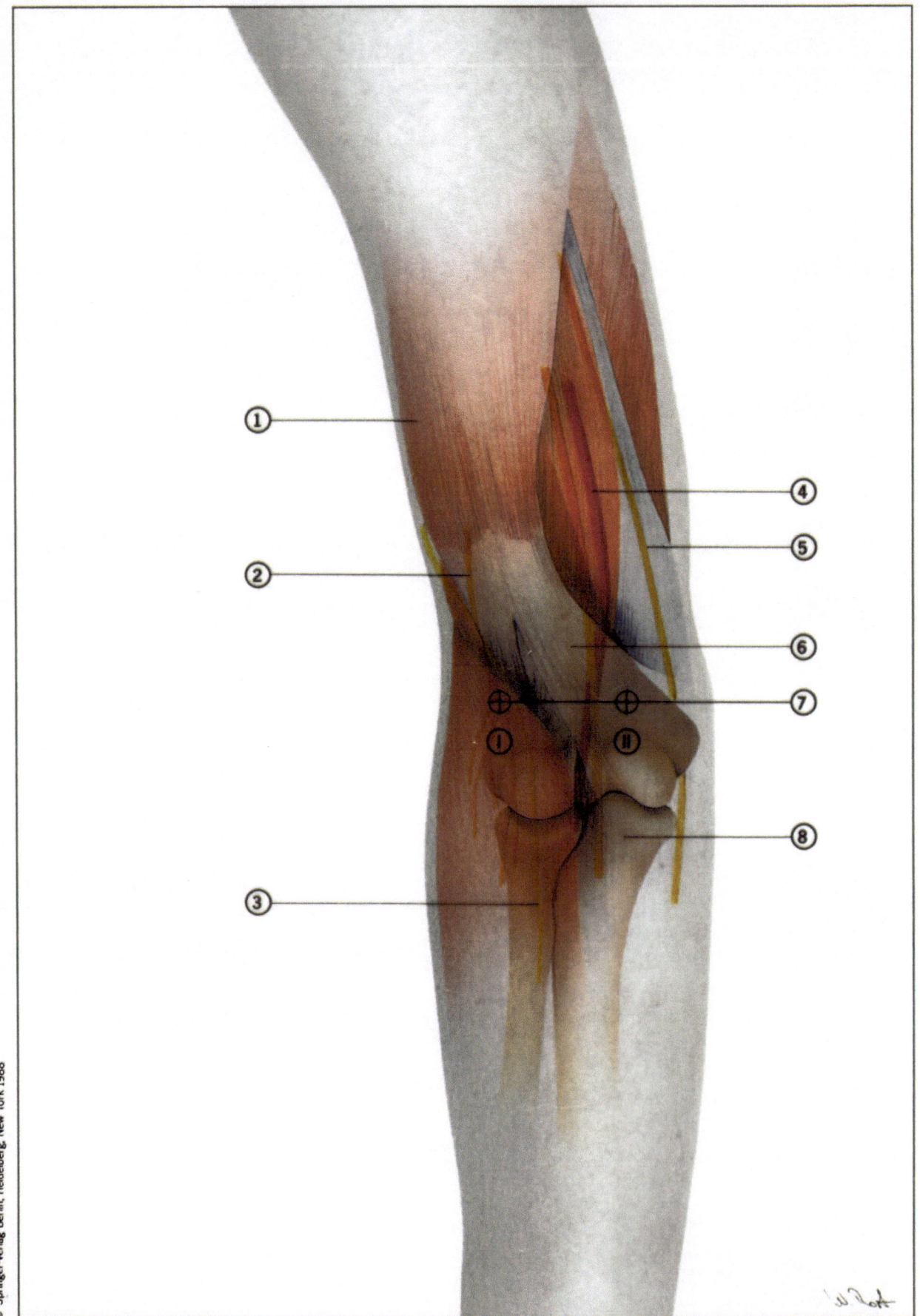

11

① Injection site for radial and musculocutaneous nerve block. ⑪ Injection site for median nerve block at elbow. ① Biceps muscle.
② Musculocutaneous nerve. ③ Radial nerve. ④ Brachial artery. ⑤ Ulnar nerve. ⑥ Tendon of biceps muscle. ⑦ Crease at the cubital fossa. ⑧ Ulna

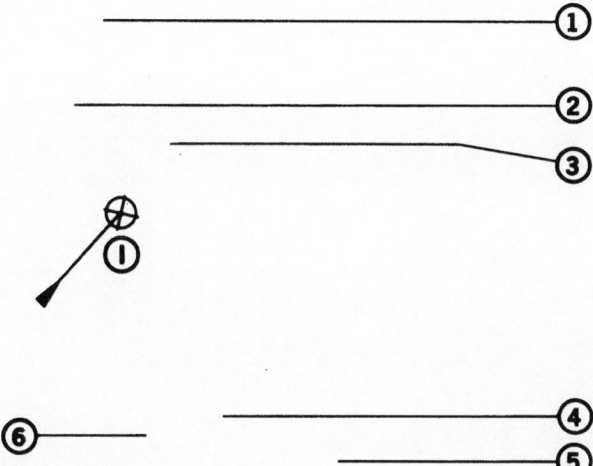

⊕ Injection site for ulnar nerve block. ① Ulna. ② Olecranon. ③ Head of radius. ④ Ulnar nerve. ⑤ Biceps muscle. ⑥ Triceps muscle

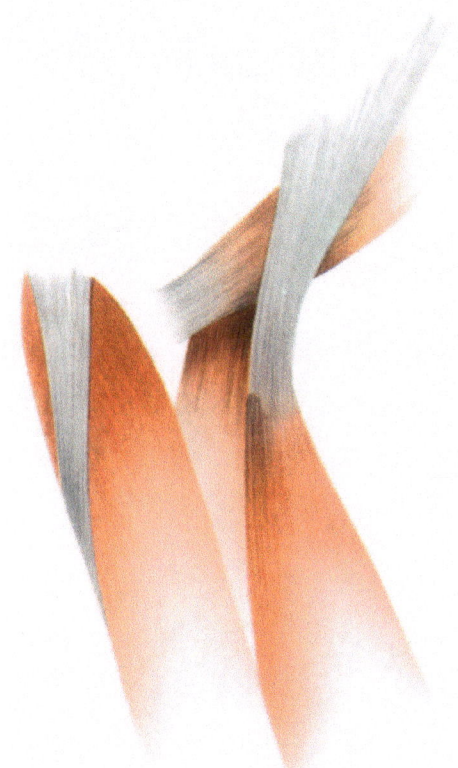

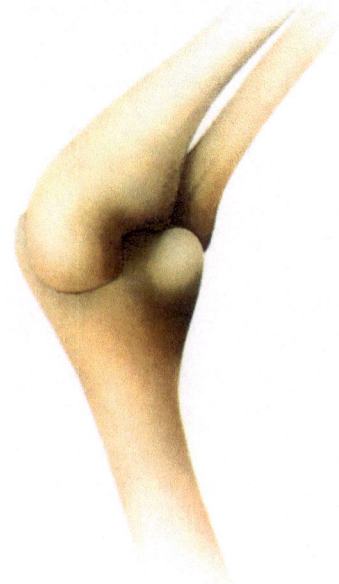

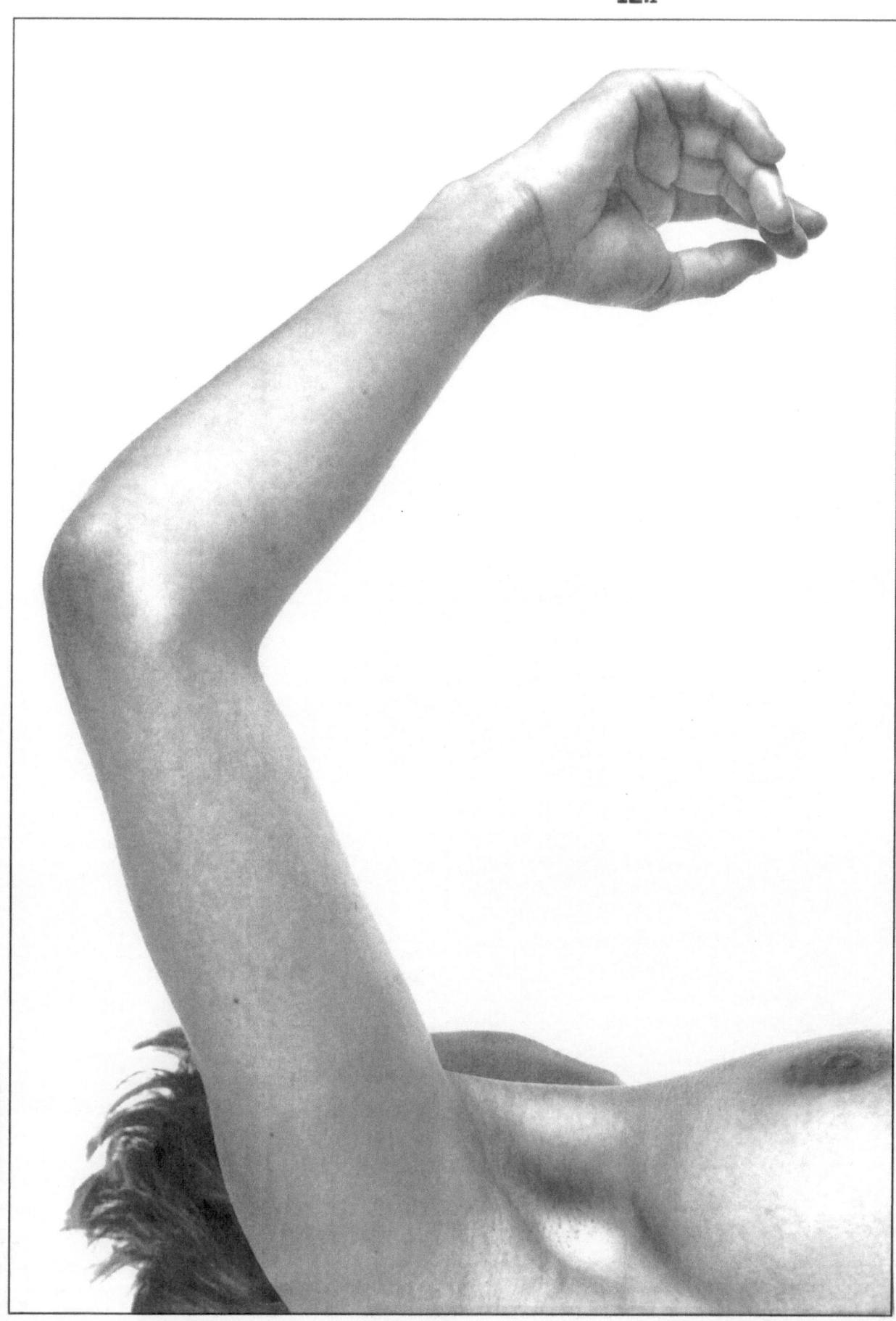

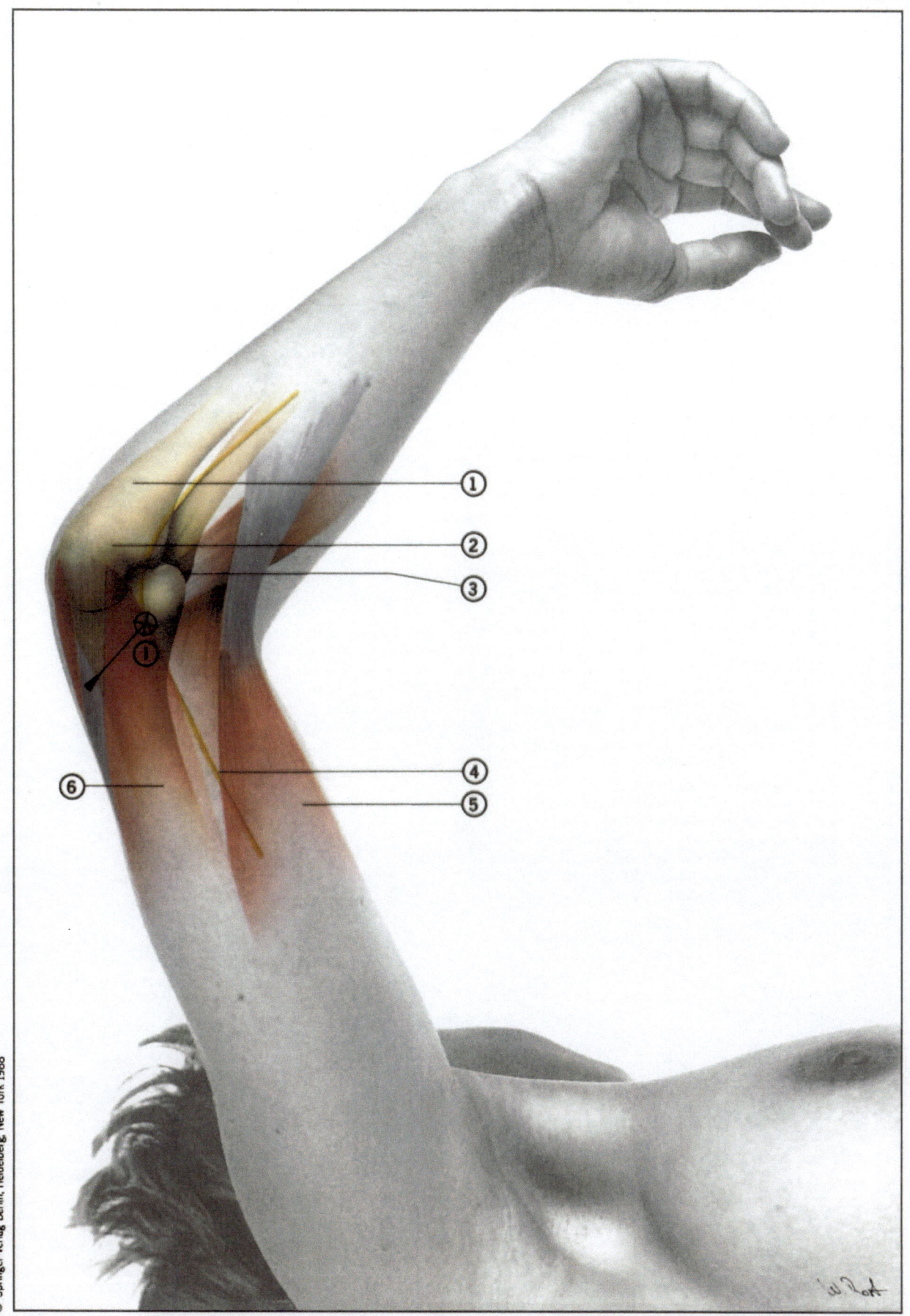

12

① Injection site for ulnar nerve block. ① Ulna. ② Olecranon. ③ Head of radius. ④ Ulnar nerve. ⑤ Biceps muscle. ⑥ Triceps muscle

© Springer-Verlag Berlin, Heidelberg, New York 1988

① Injection site for ulnar nerve block at wrist. ⑪ Injection site for median nerve block. ① Tendon of palmaris longus muscle. ② Styloid process of ulna. ③ Ulnar nerve with ulnar artery. ④ Ulna. ⑤ Median nerve. ⑥ Radial artery. ⑦ Tendon of flexor carpi radialis muscle

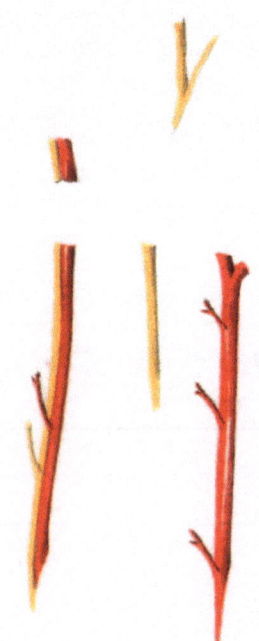

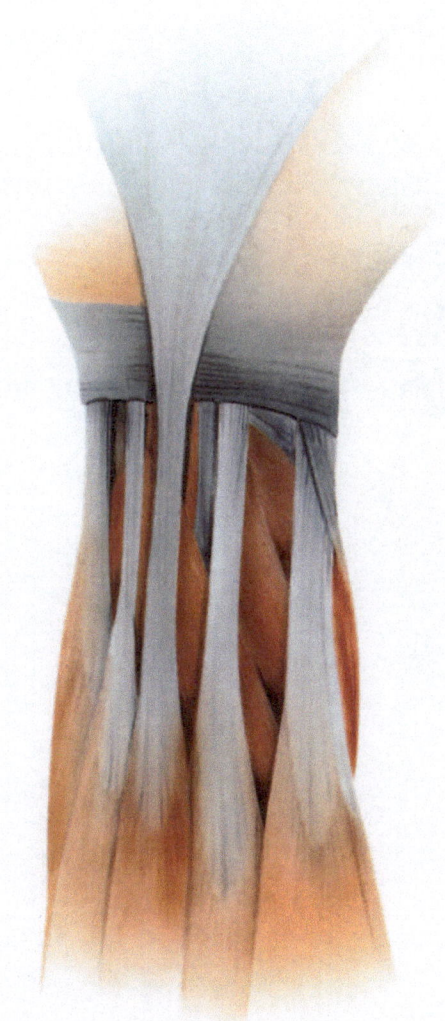

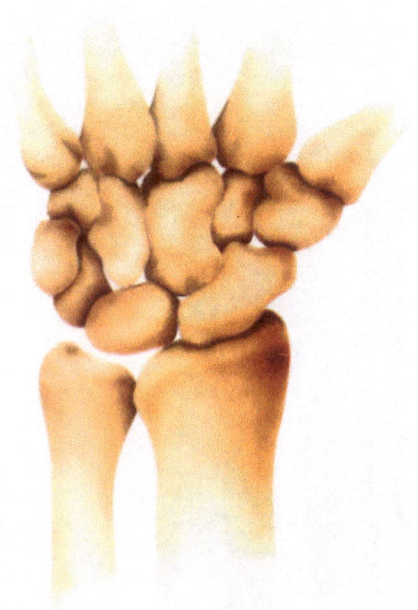

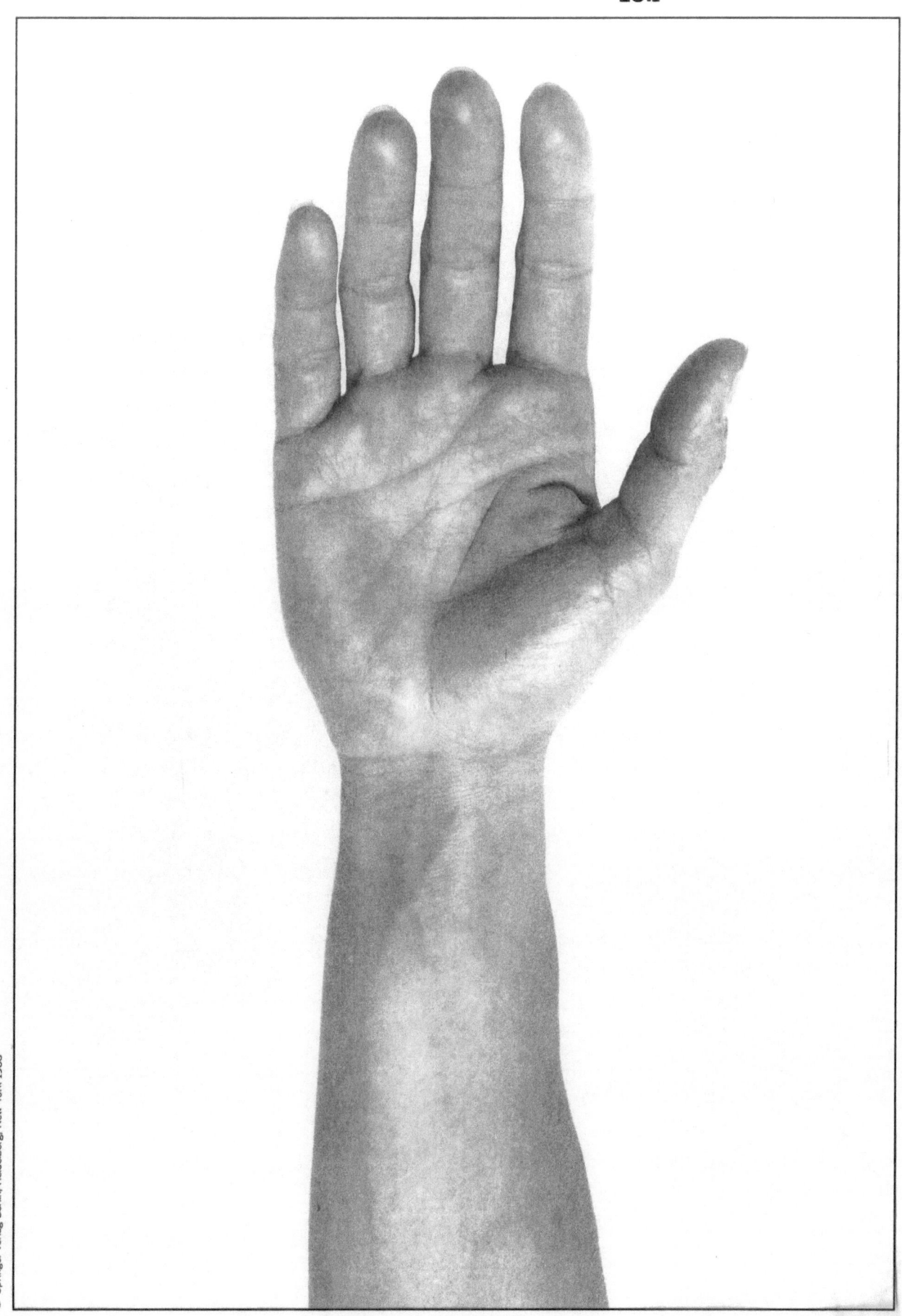

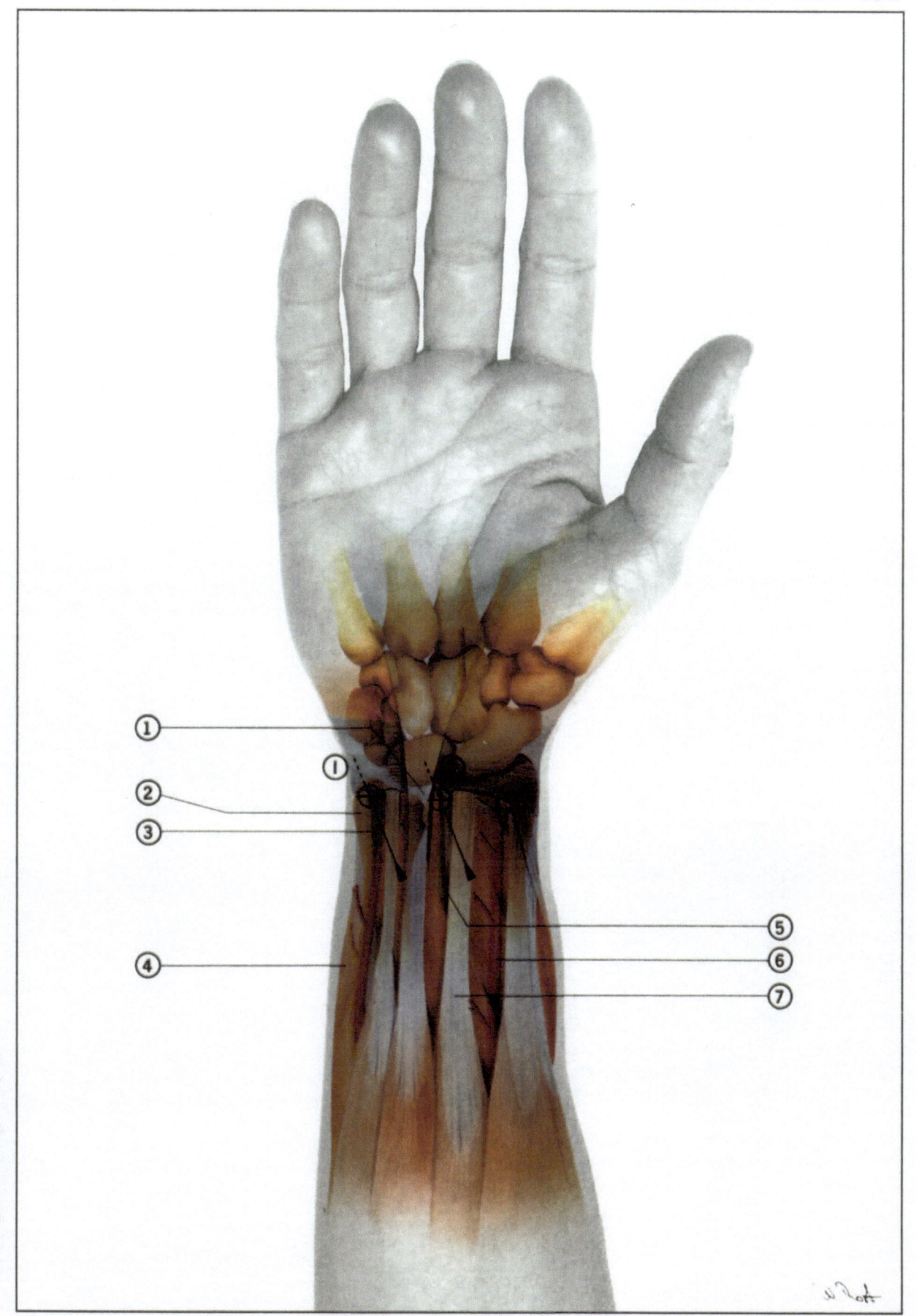

① Injection site for ulnar nerve block at wrist. ⑪ Injection site for median nerve block. ① Tendon of palmaris longus muscle. ② Styloid process of ulna. ③ Ulnar nerve with ulnar artery. ④ Ulna. ⑤ Median nerve. ⑥ Radial artery. ⑦ Tendon of flexor carpi radialis muscle

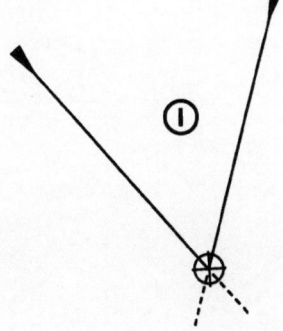

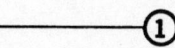

① Injection site for radial nerve block at wrist. ① Superficial radial nerve

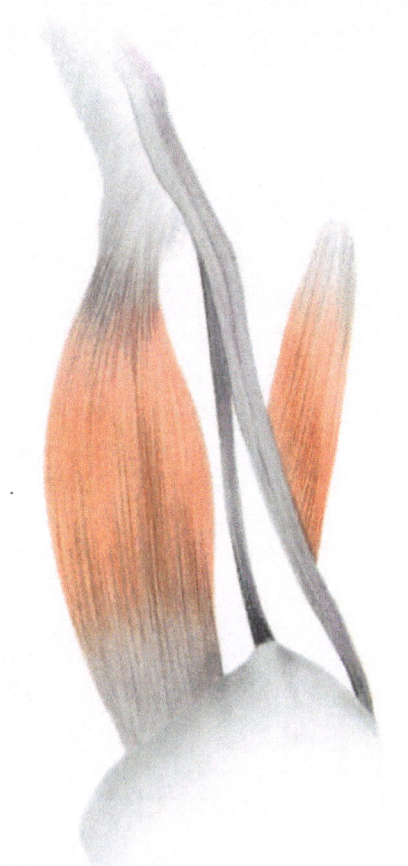

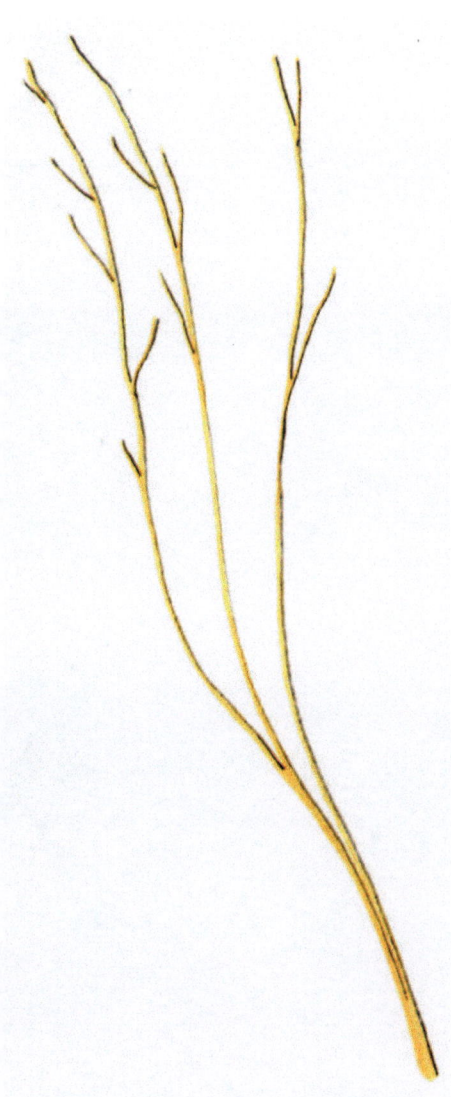

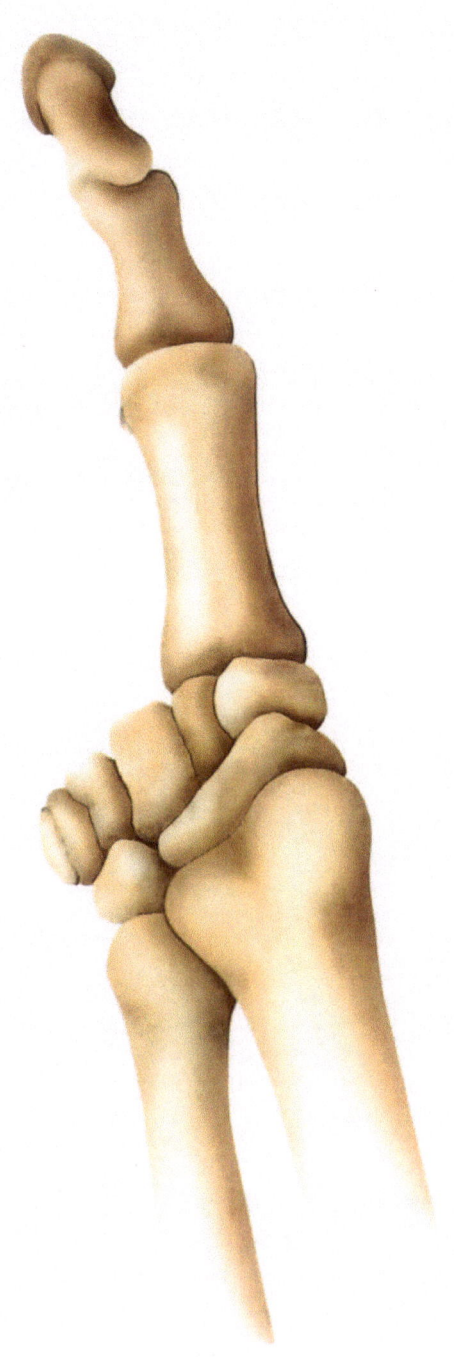

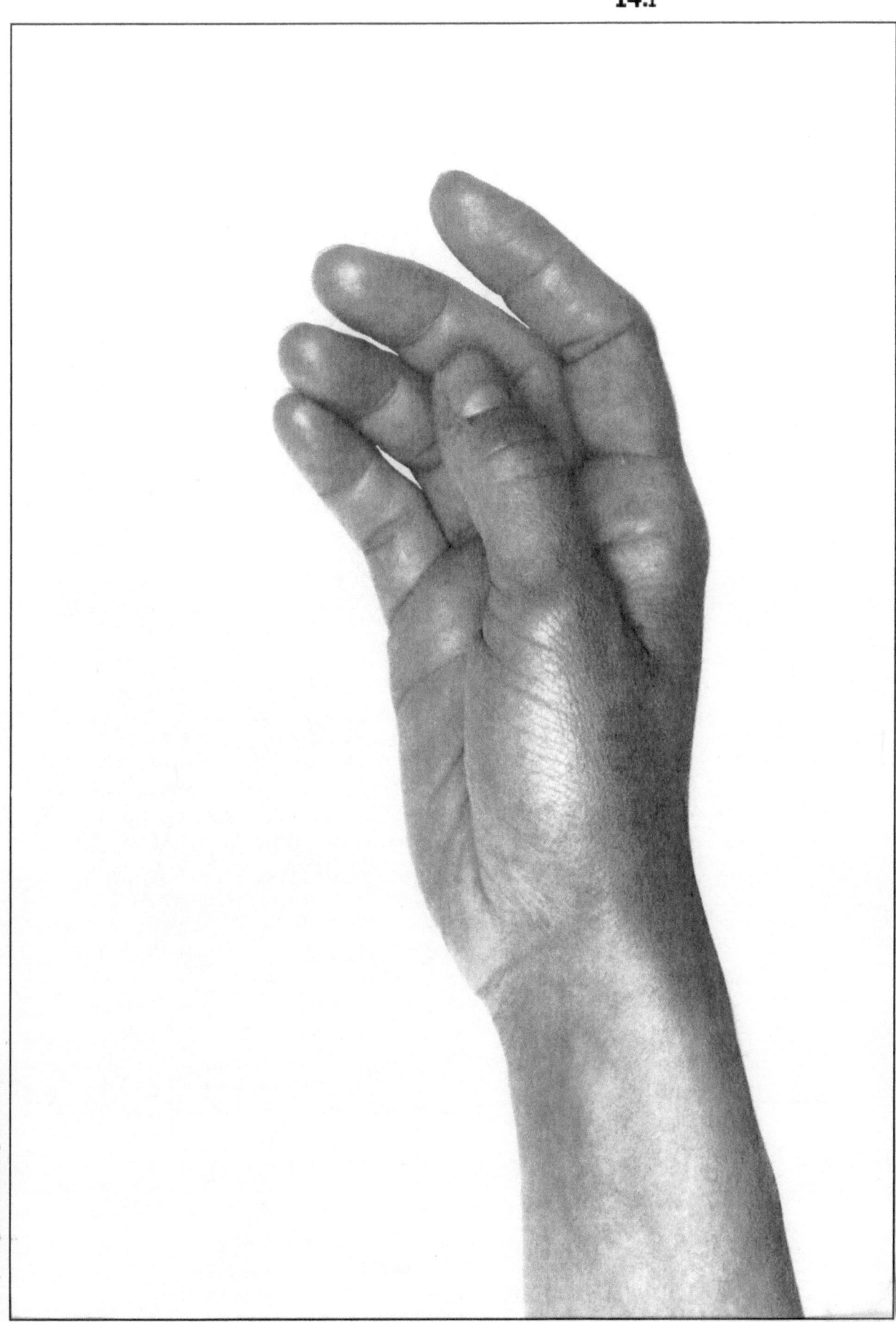

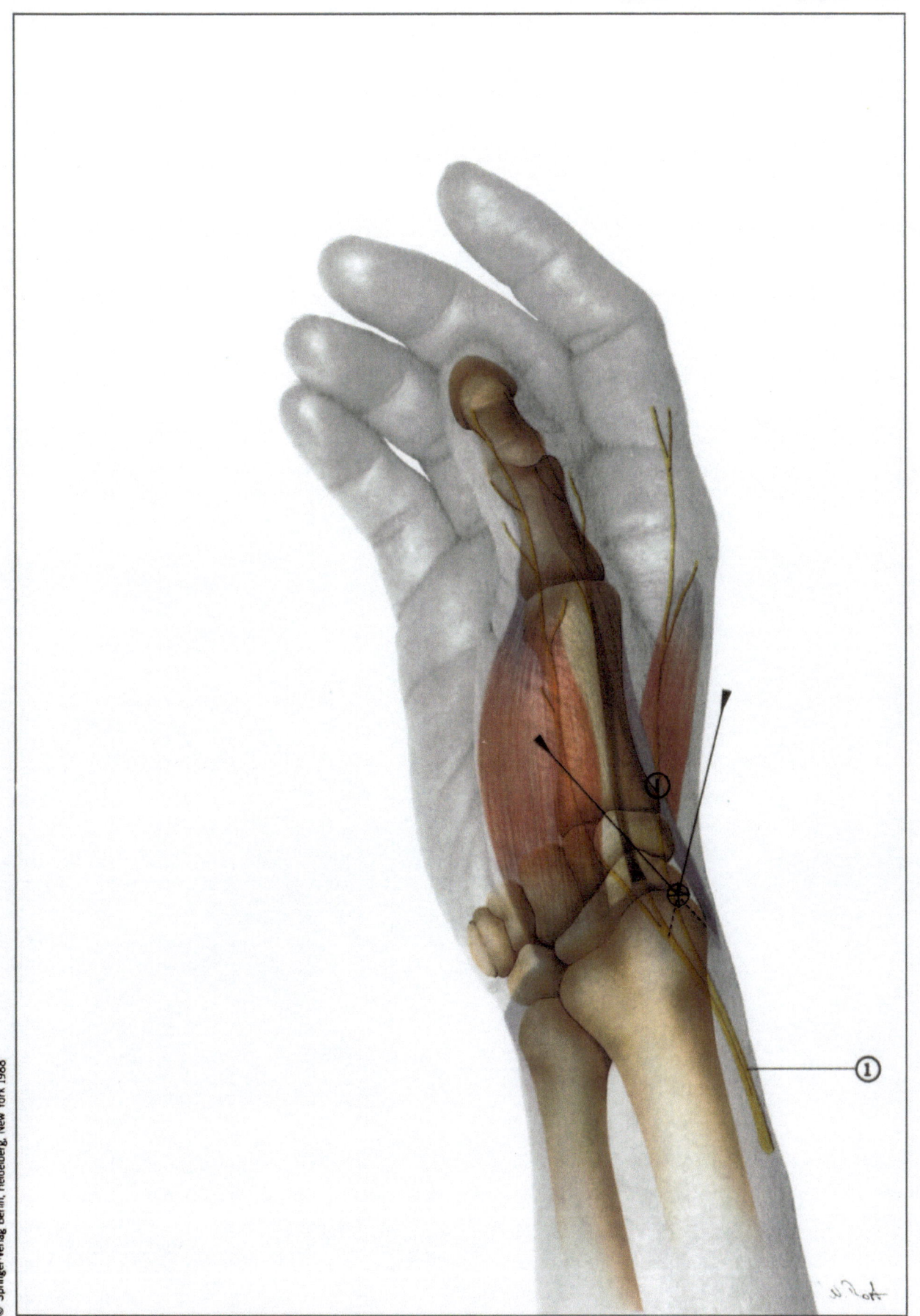

① Injection site for radial nerve block at wrist. ① Superficial radial nerve

① Injection sites for metacarpal nerve block. ⑪ Injection sites into the web space between the digits. ⑪⑪ Injection sites at base of digits. ① Dorsal digital nerve. ② Dorsal branches of ulnar nerve. ③ Dorsal interosseous muscle. ④ Radial nerve

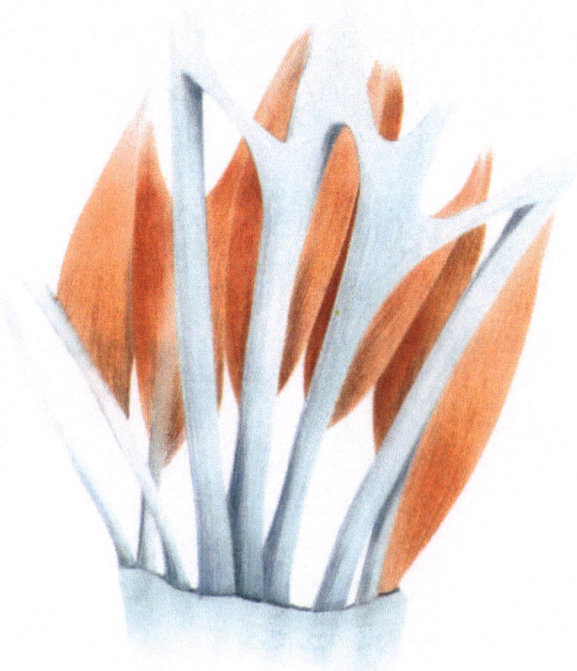

15.3

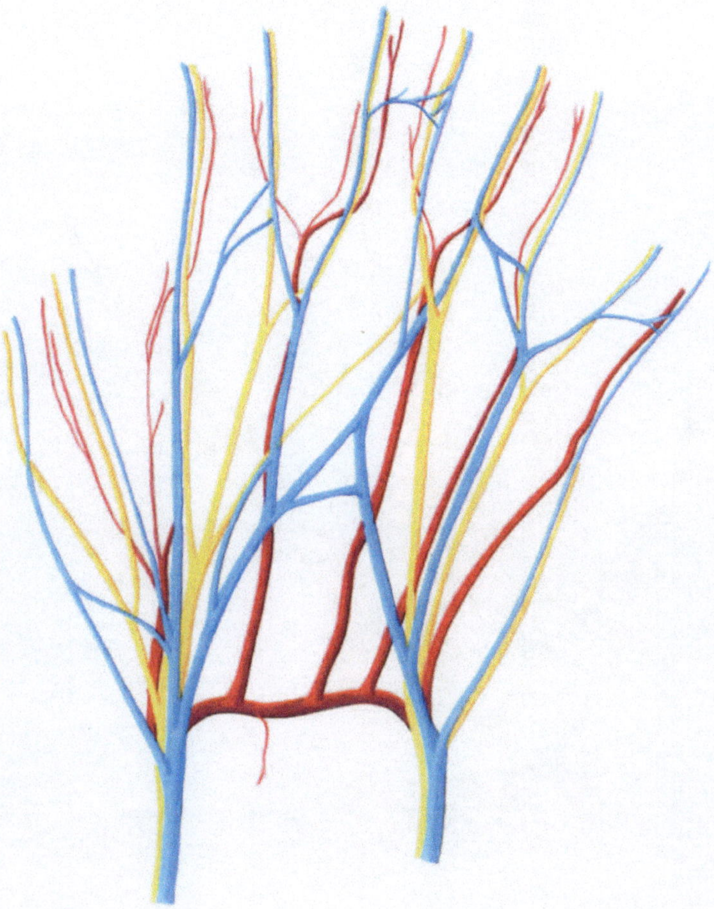

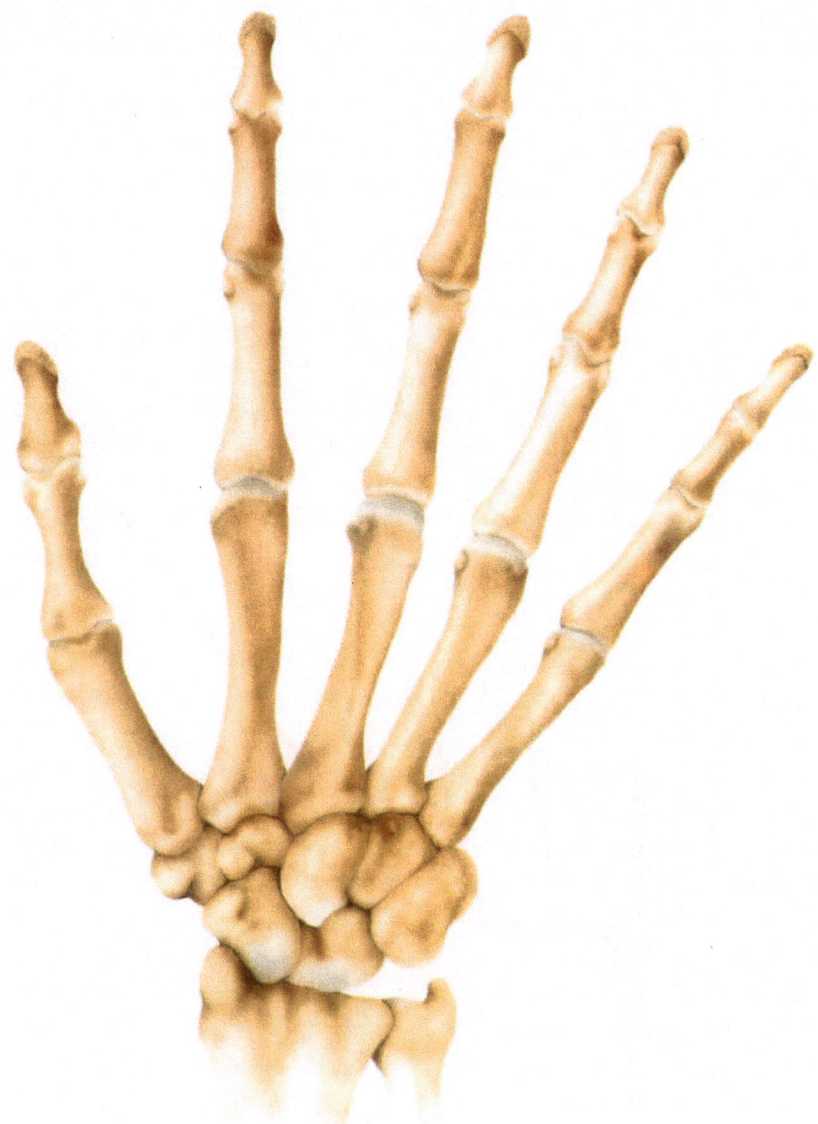

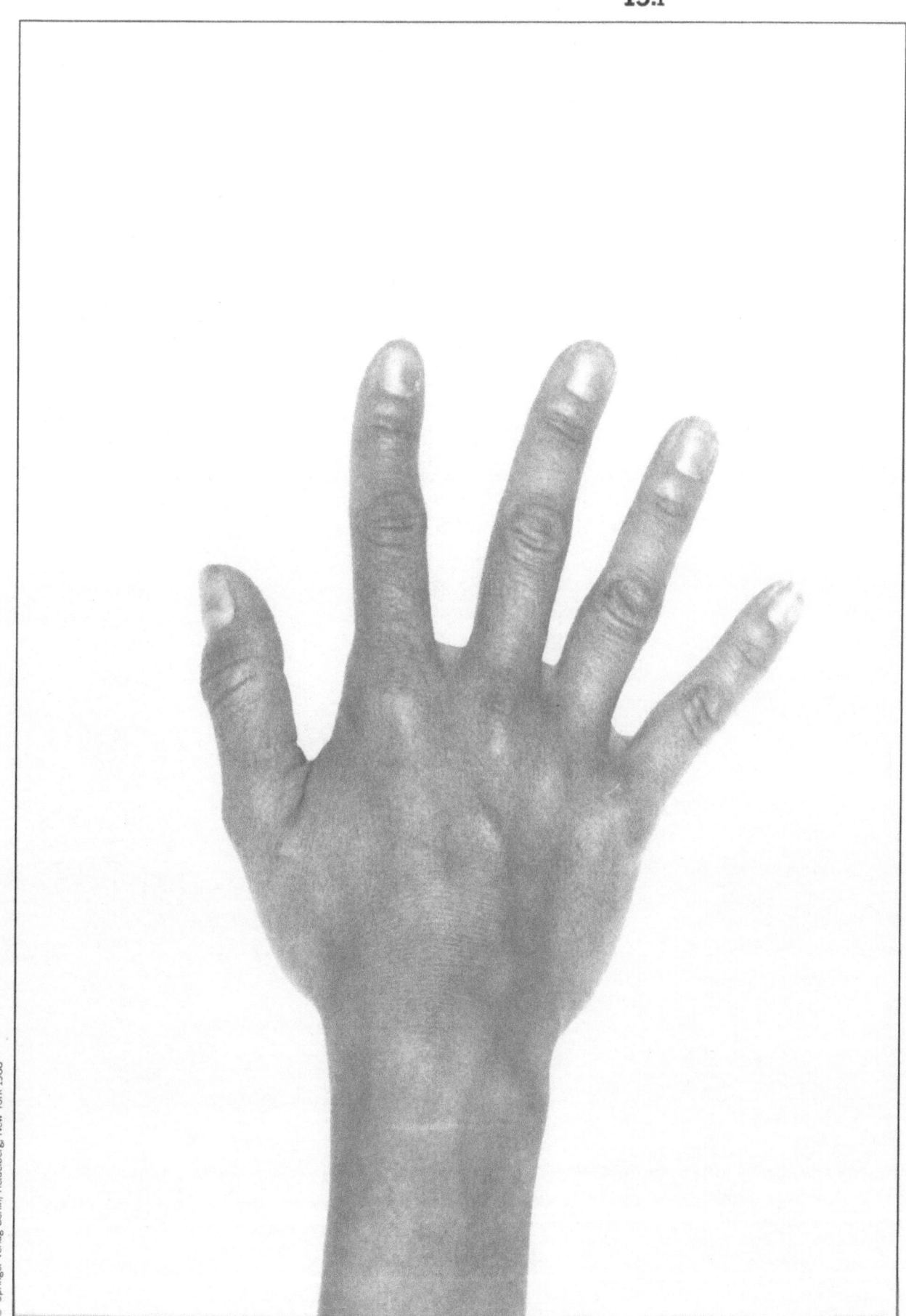

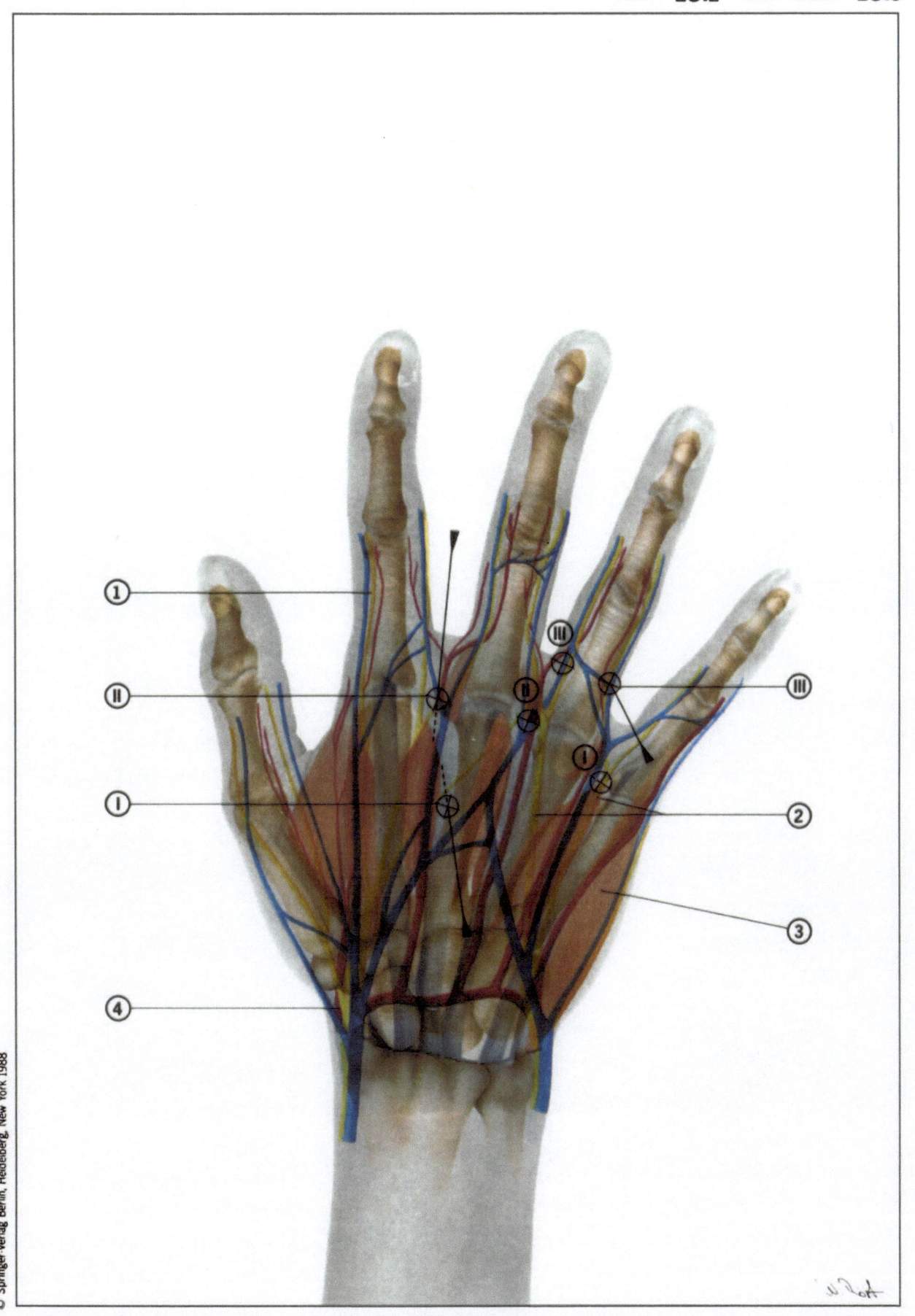

① Injection sites for metacarpal nerve block. ② Injection sites into the web space between the digits. ③ Injection sites at base of digits. ① Dorsal digital nerve. ② Dorsal branches of ulnar nerve. ③ Dorsal interosseous muscle. ④ Radial nerve

B

④
③
A - ⊛ - - - - - - - - - - - - - - - - - - A

⑤

①

②

①

B

① Injection site for lumbar plexus block. A ----A: Intercristal line between iliac crests marking L3–4 interspace. B----B: Line through posterior superior iliac spine parallel to spinous processes. ① Sciatic nerve. ② Posterior superior iliac spine. ③ Formation of lumbar plexus in psoas muscle. ④ Psoas muscle. ⑤ Transverse process of L4

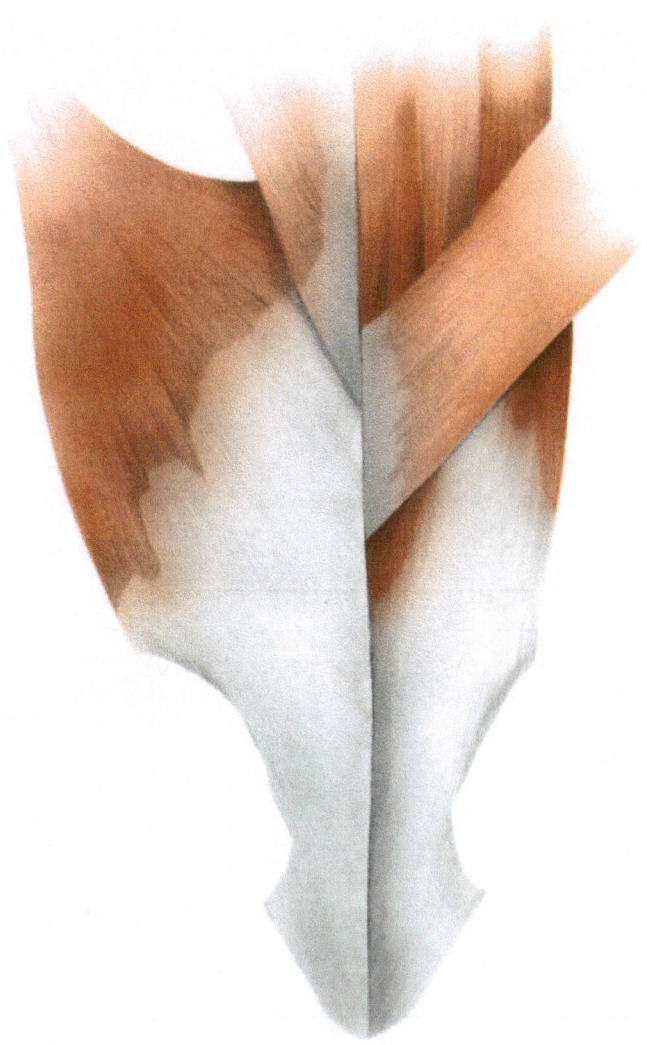

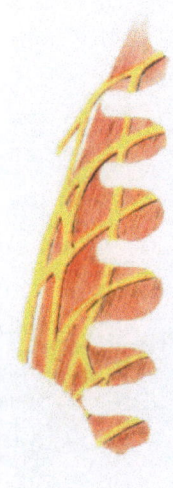

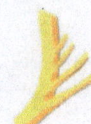

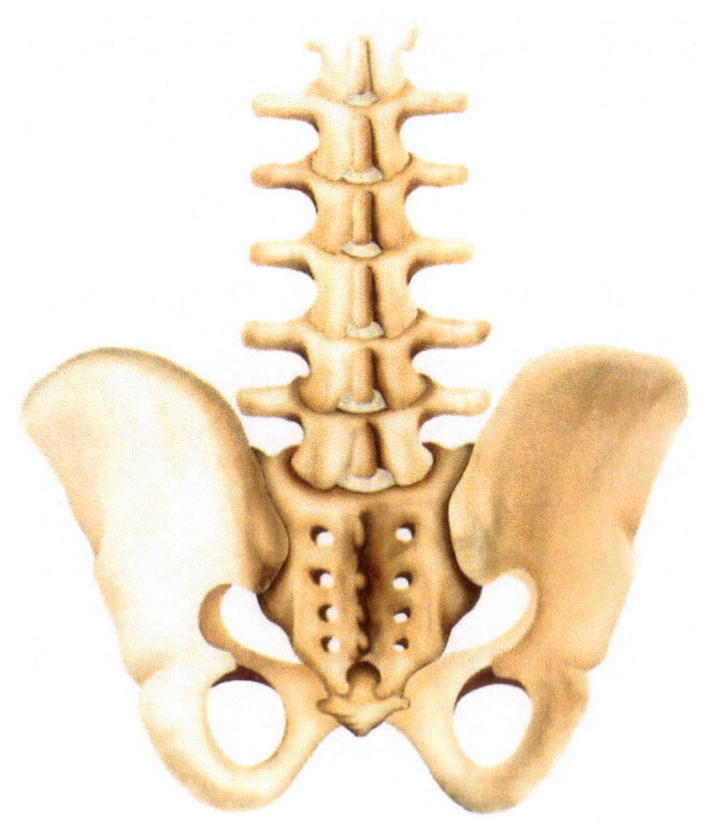

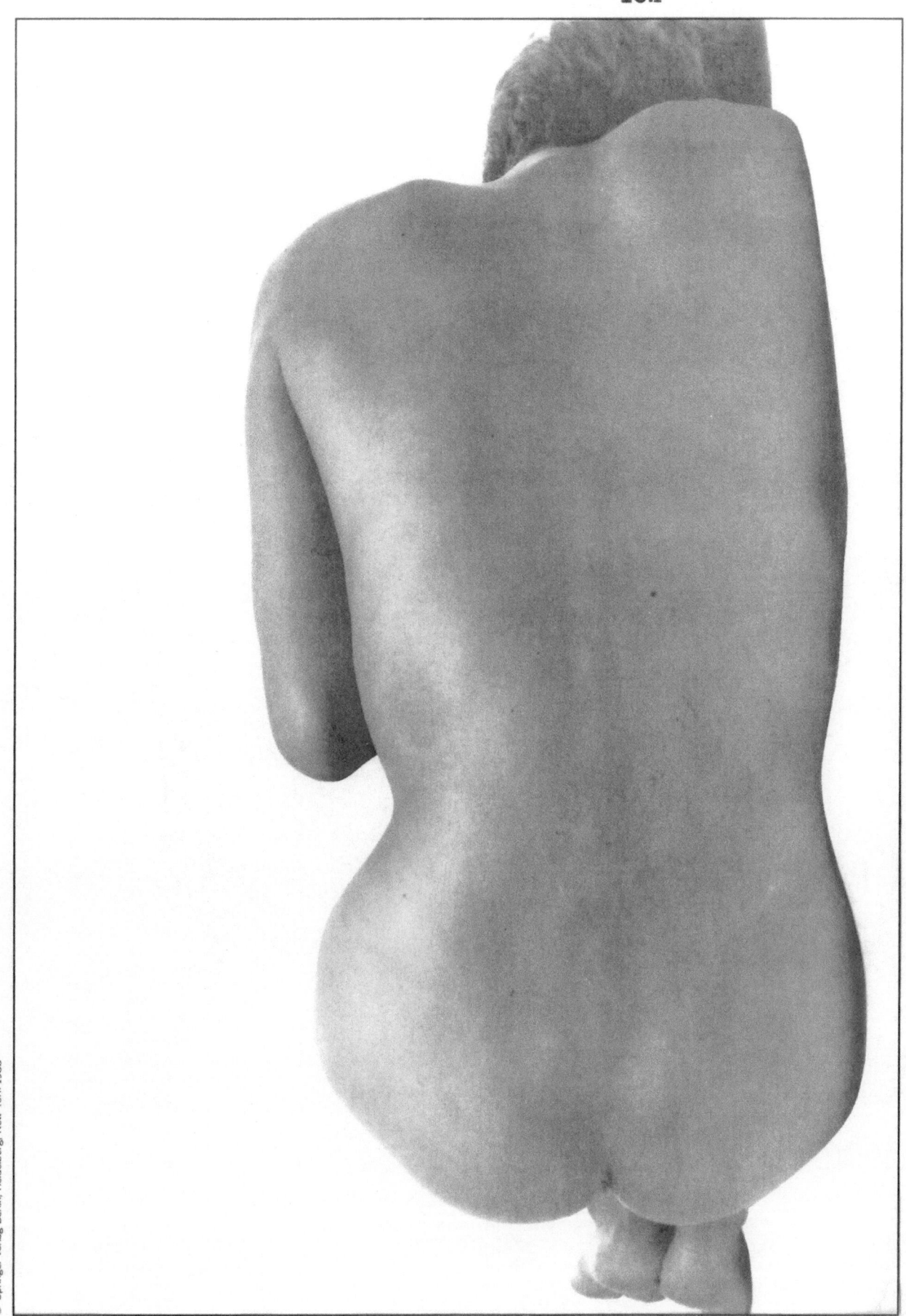

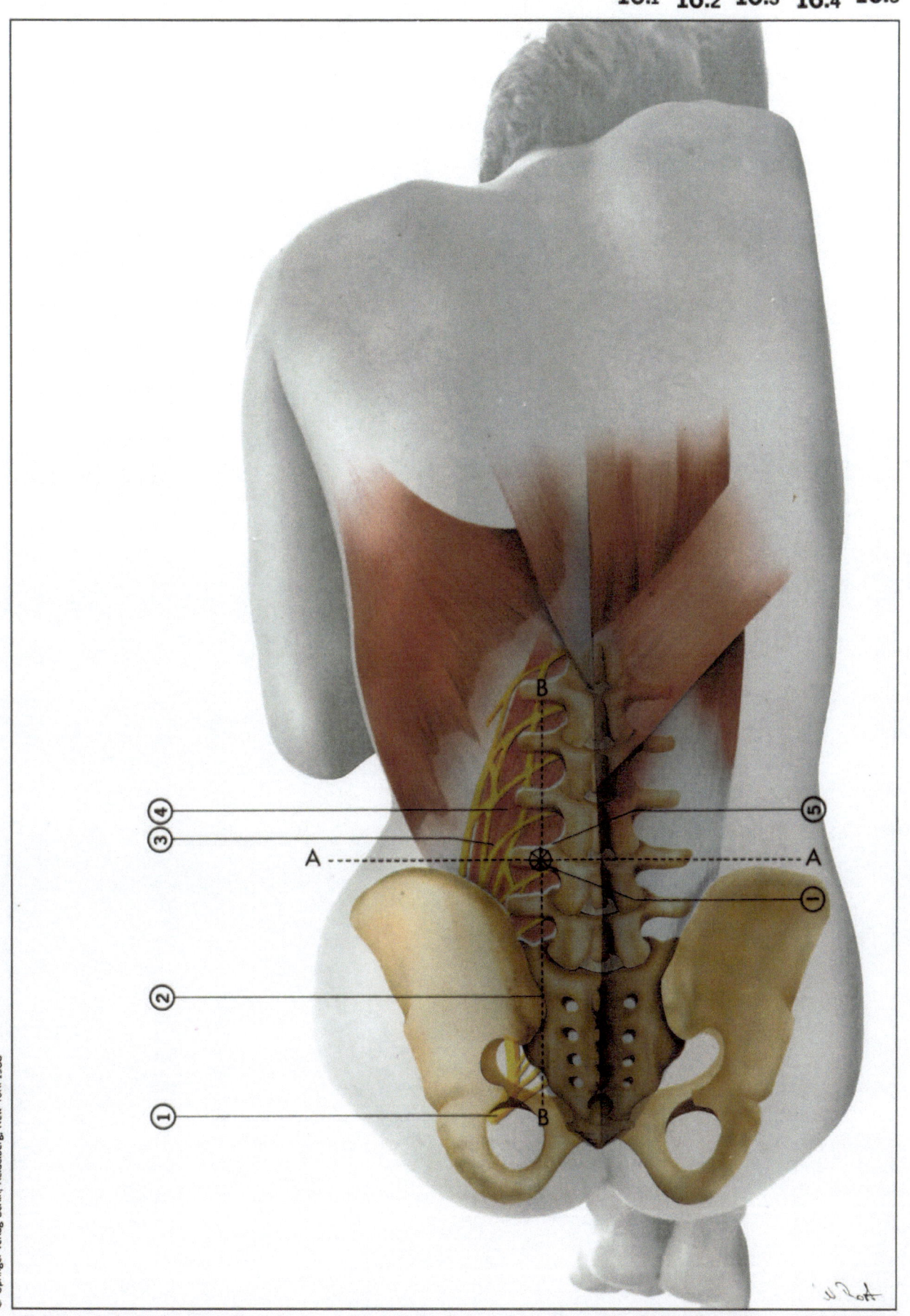

① Injection site for lumbar plexus block. A – – – – A: Intercristal line between iliac crests marking L3–4 interspace. B – – – – B: Line through posterior superior iliac spine parallel to spinous processes. ① Sciatic nerve. ② Posterior superior iliac spine. ③ Formation of lumbar plexus in psoas muscle. ④ Psoas muscle. ⑤ Transverse process of L4

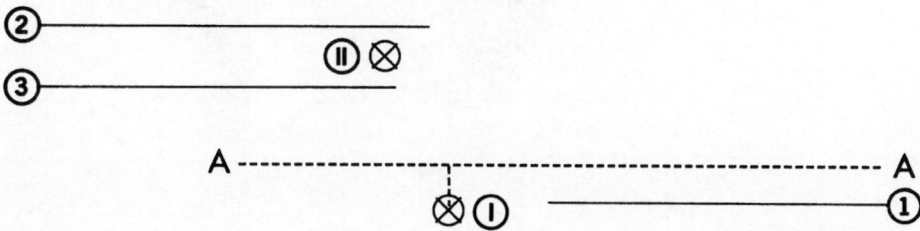

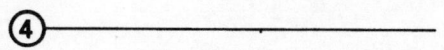

① Injection site for psoas compartment block. ⑪ Alternative injection site for psoas compartment block. A – – – – A: Intercristal line joining iliac crests. ① Spinous process of L4. ② Psoas muscle. ③ Formation of lumbar plexus in psoas muscle. ④ Sciatic nerve

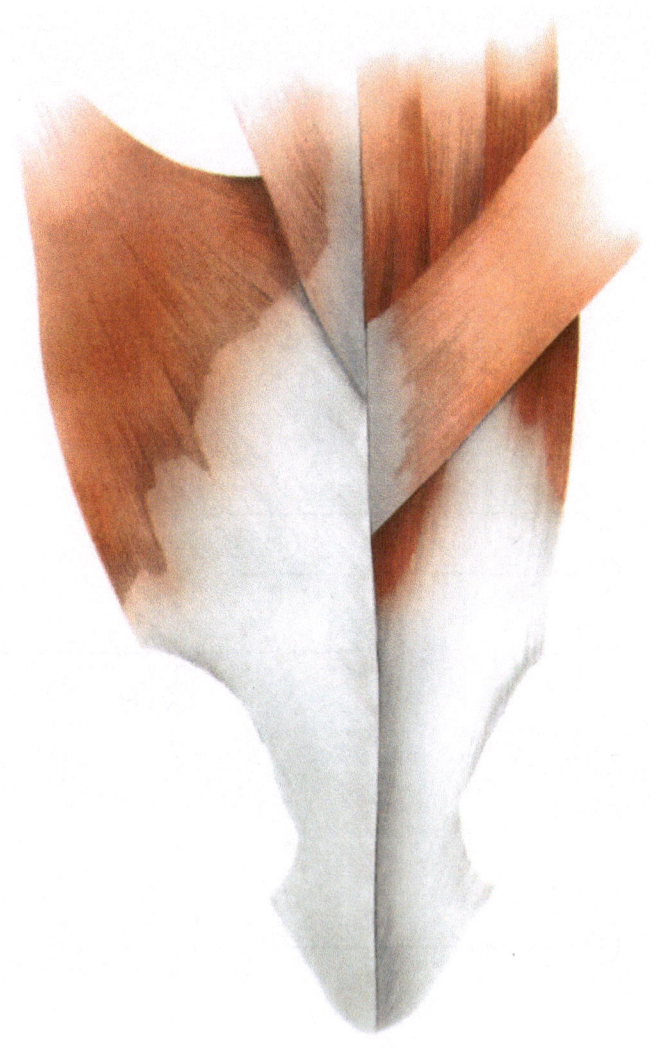

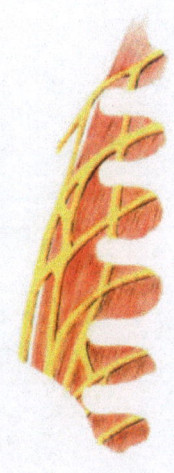

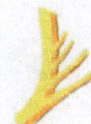

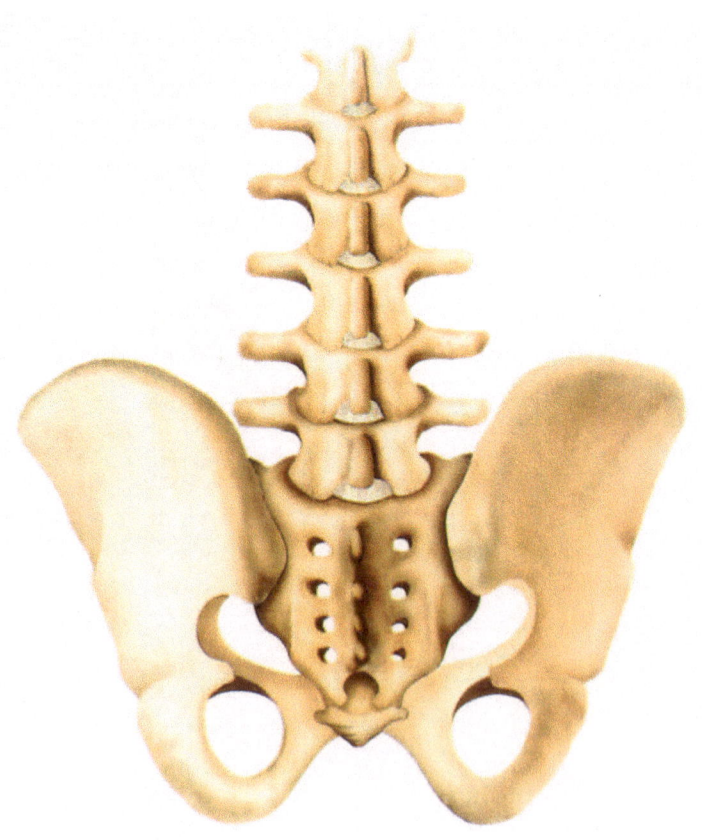

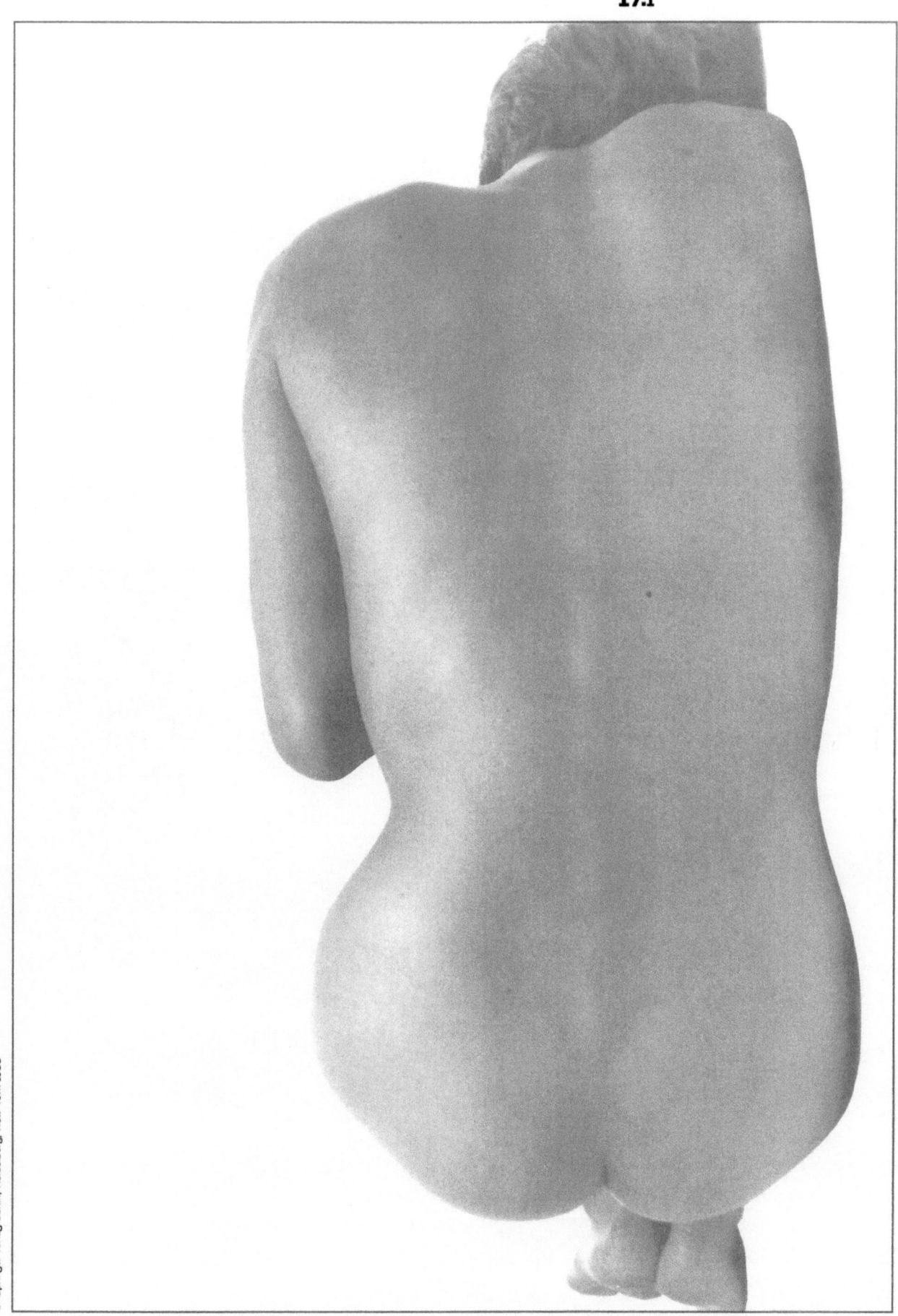

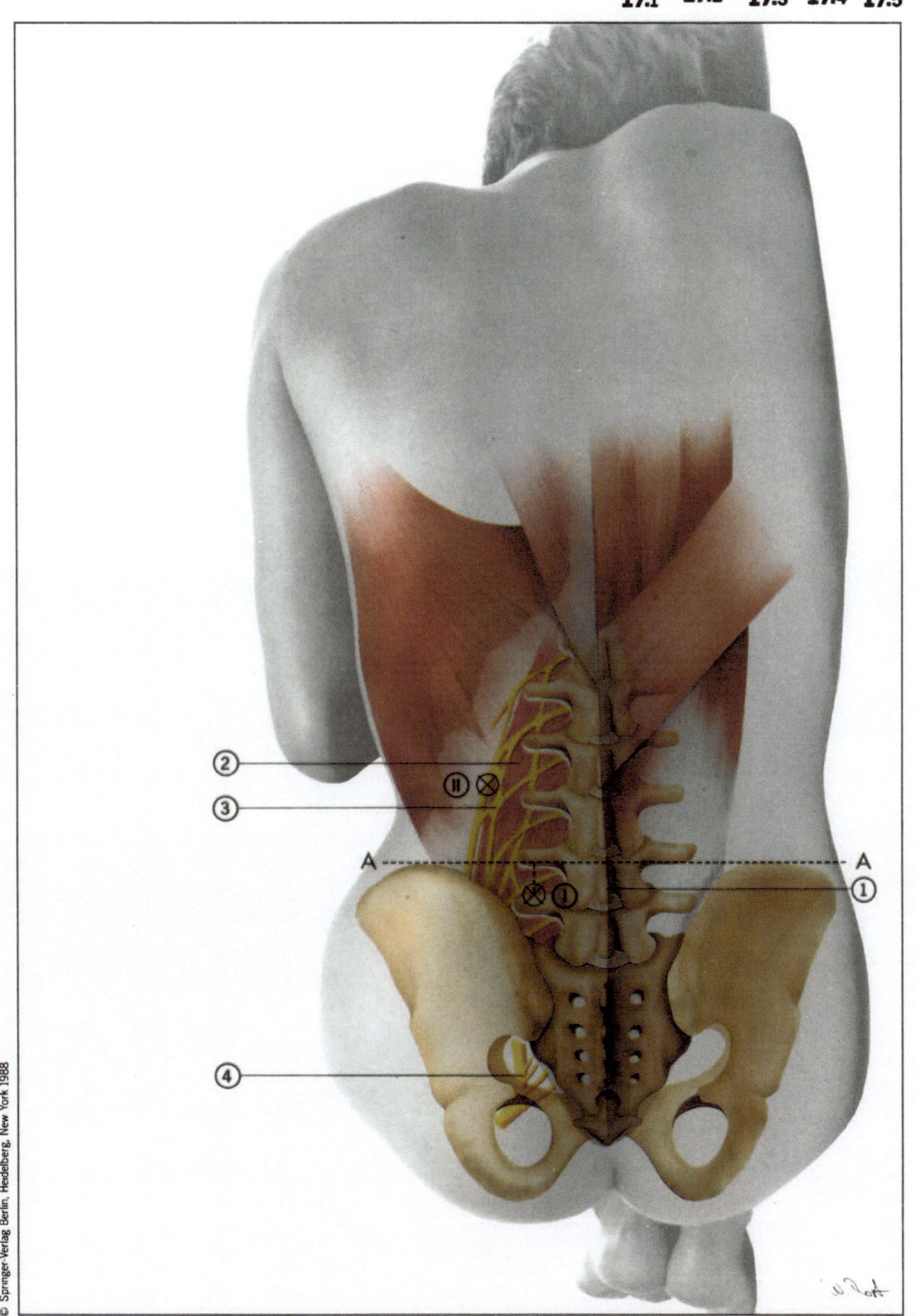

① Injection site for psoas compartment block. ⑪ Alternative injection site for psoas compartment block. A ‒‒‒‒ A: Intercristal line joining iliac crests. ① Spinous process of L4. ② Psoas muscle. ③ Formation of lumbar plexus in psoas muscle. ④ Sciatic nerve

① Injection site for sciatic nerve block (posterior approach). A – – – – A: Line joining posterior superior iliac spine and greater trochanter. A – – – – B: Line joining sacral hiatus and greater trochanter. C – – – – C: Line joining A – – A and A – – B drawn perpendicularly from midpoint of A – – A. ① Greater trochanter. ② Sciatic nerve. ③ Posterior superior iliac spine. ④ Sacral hiatus

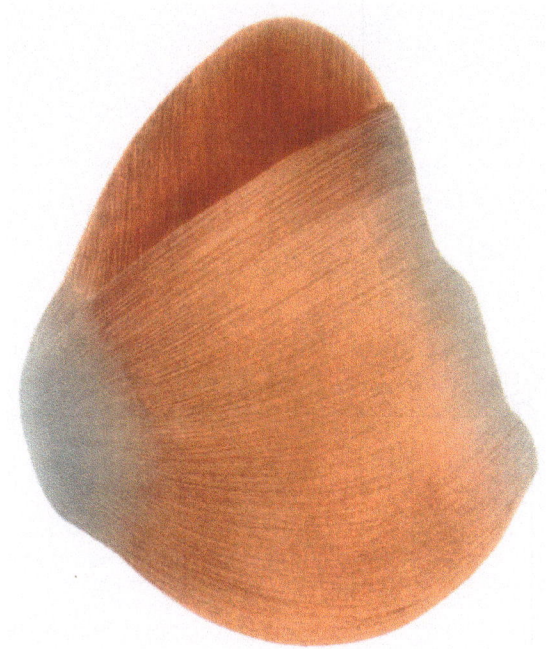

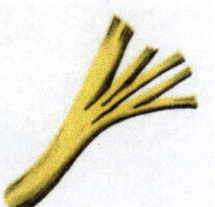

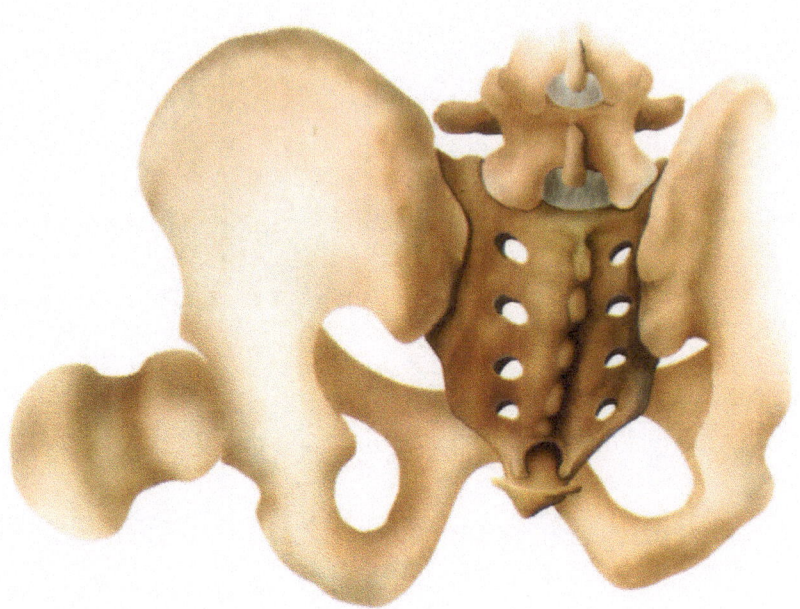

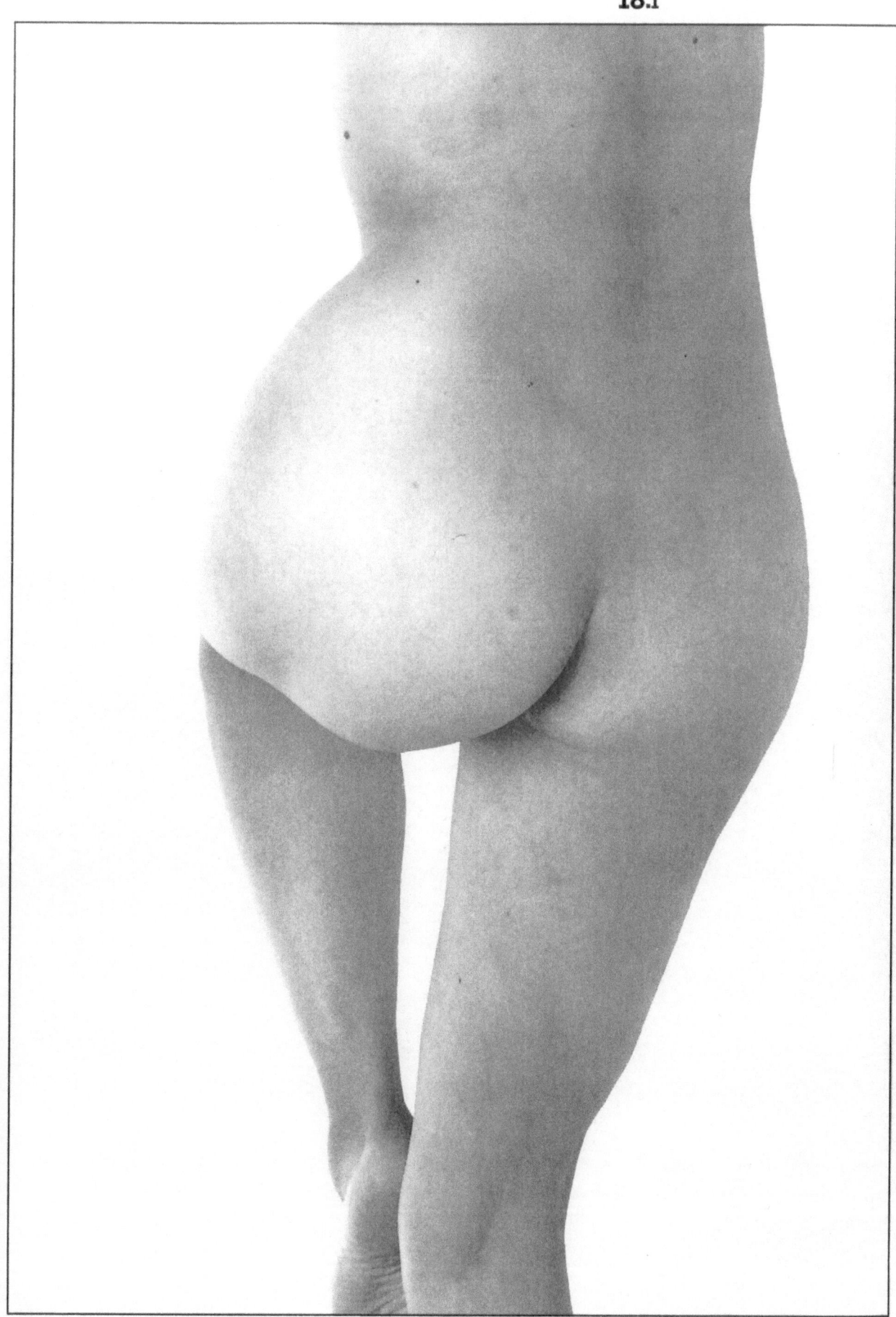

Sciatic Nerve Block: Posterior Approach

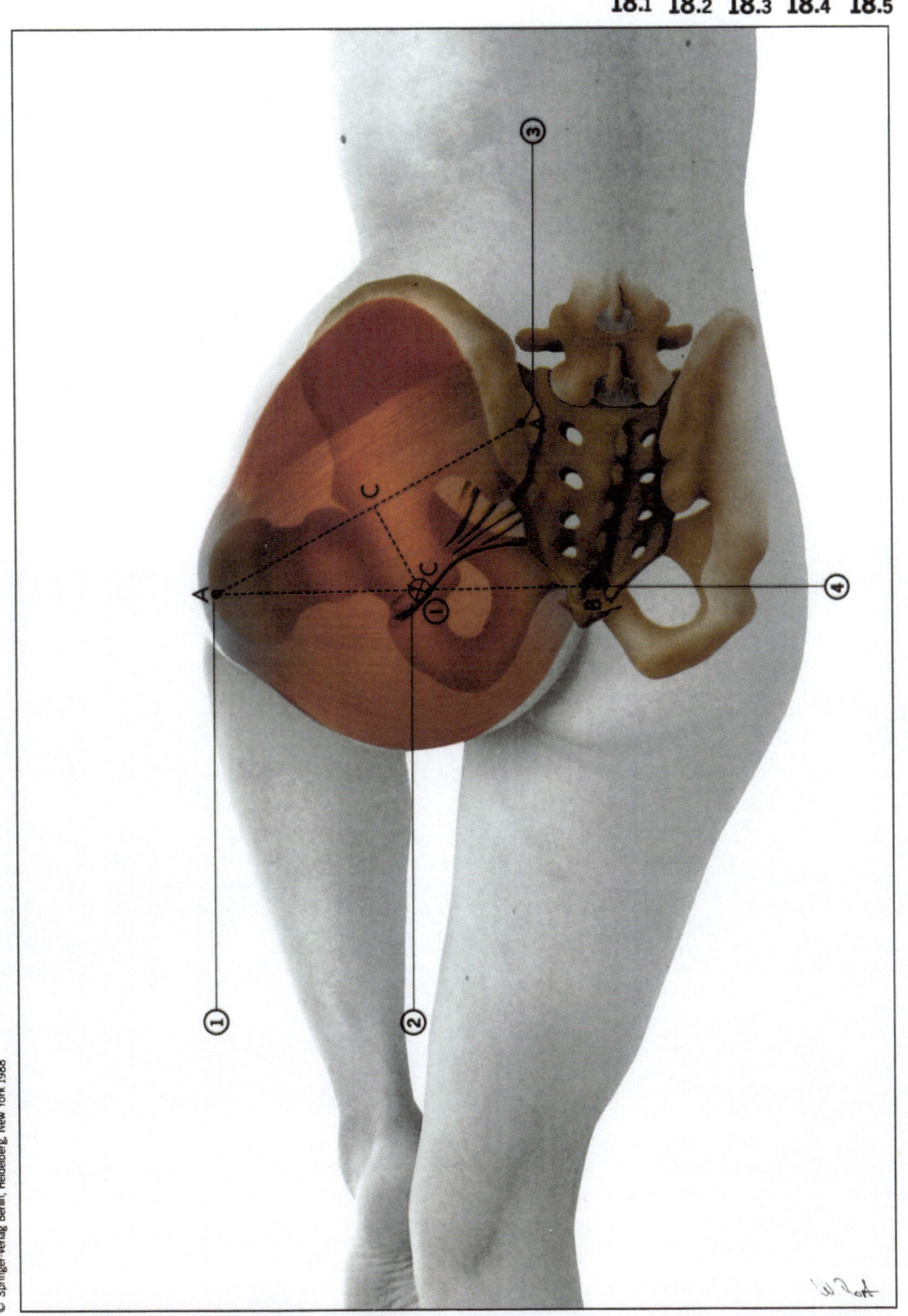

① Injection site for sciatic nerve block (posterior approach). A – – – – A: Line joining posterior superior iliac spine and greater trochanter. A – – – – B: Line joining sacral hiatus and greater trochanter. C – – – – C: Line joining A – – A and A – – B drawn perpendicularly from midpoint of A – – A. ① Greater trochanter. ② Sciatic nerve. ③ Posterior superior iliac spine. ④ Sacral hiatus

① A
② B
① C
③ C⊕ B
C
A
④
⑤
⑥
⑦
⑧
⑨
⑩

© Springer-Verlag Berlin, Heidelberg, New York 1988

① Injection site for sciatic nerve block (supine anterior approach). A – – – – A: Line from anterior superior iliac spine to pubic tubercle.
B – – – – B: line from greater to lesser trochanter running parallel to line A – – A. C – – – – C: Line drawn perpendicular to A – – A and B – – B
at medial third of A – – A. ① Anterior superior iliac spine. ② Greater trochanter. ③ Lesser trochanter. ④ Femoral nerve. ⑤ Femoral artery.
⑥ Femoral vein. ⑦ Pubic tubercle. ⑧ Sciatic nerve. ⑨ Adductor longus muscle. ⑩ Sartorius muscle

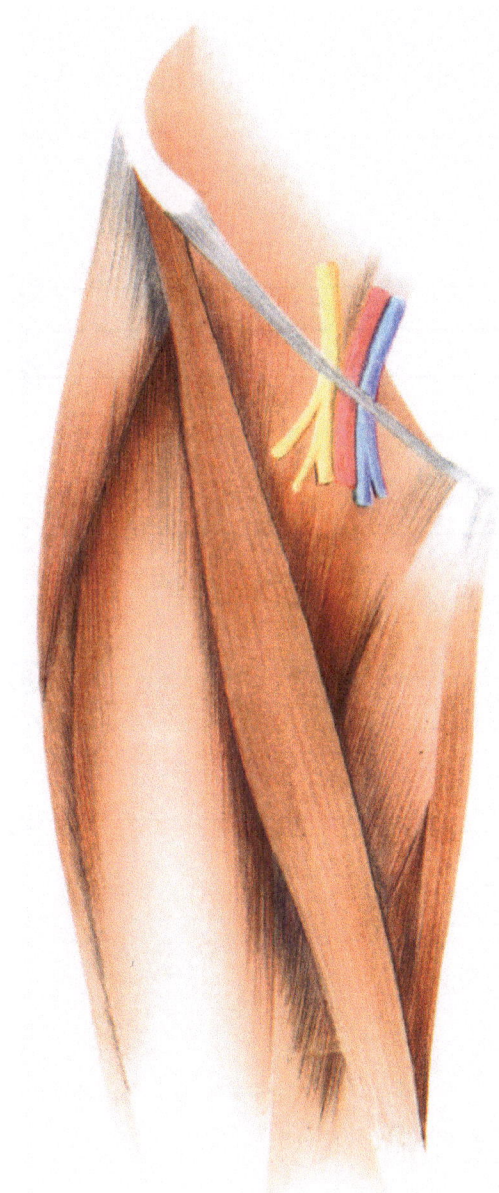

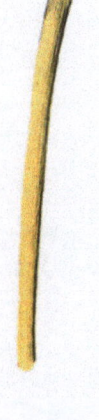

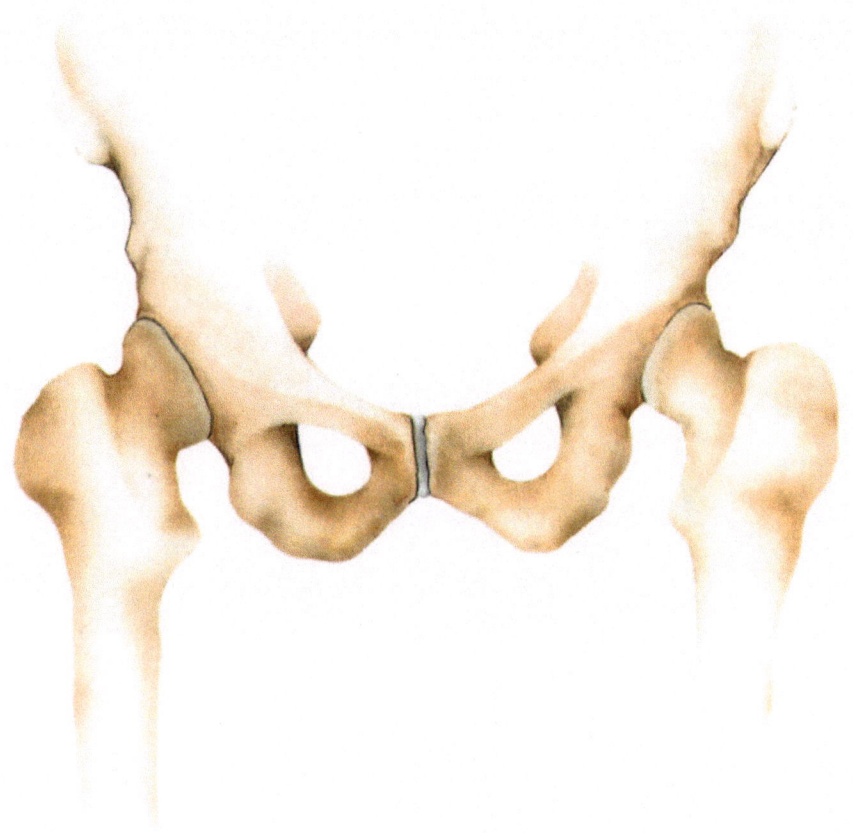

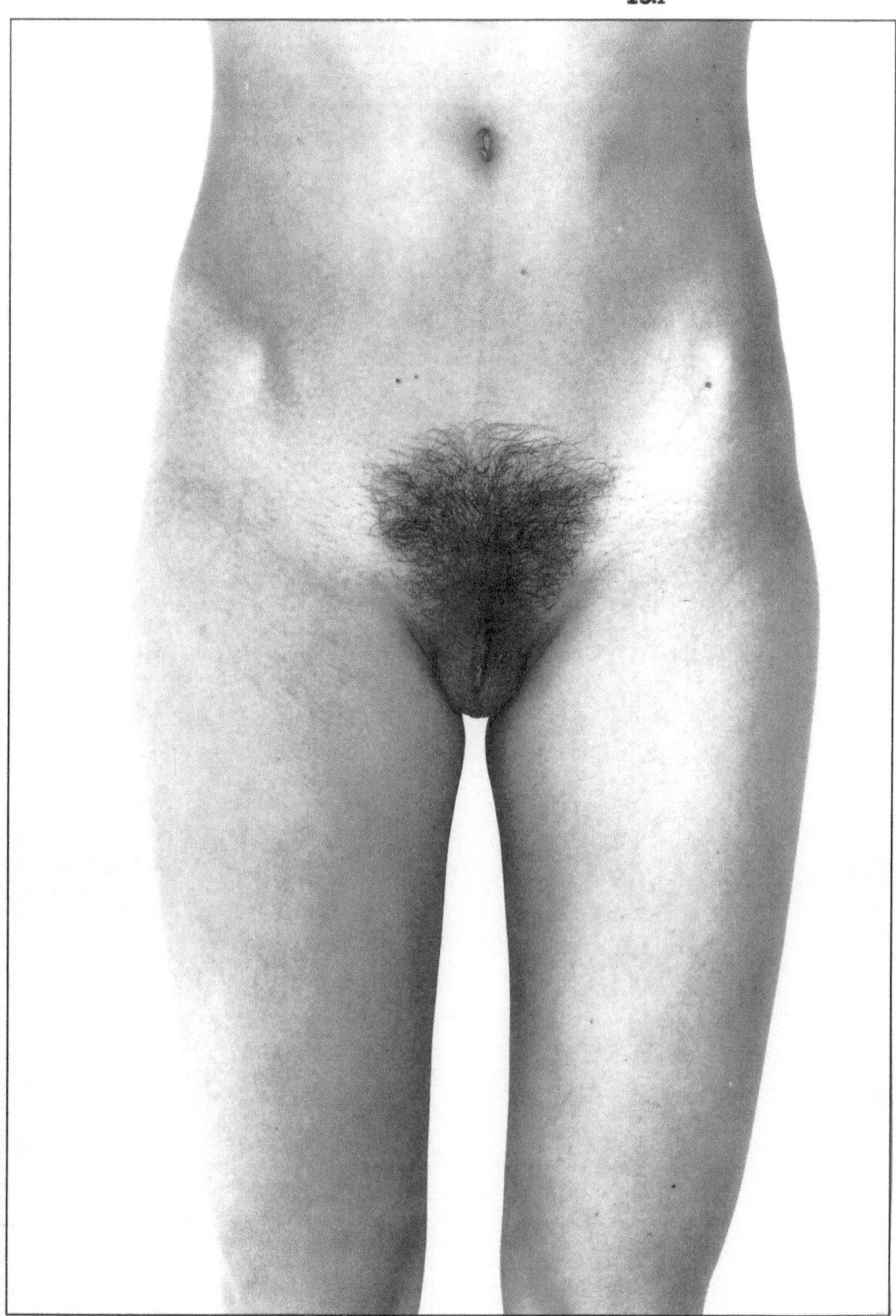

Sciatic Nerve Block: Supine Anterior Approach

19

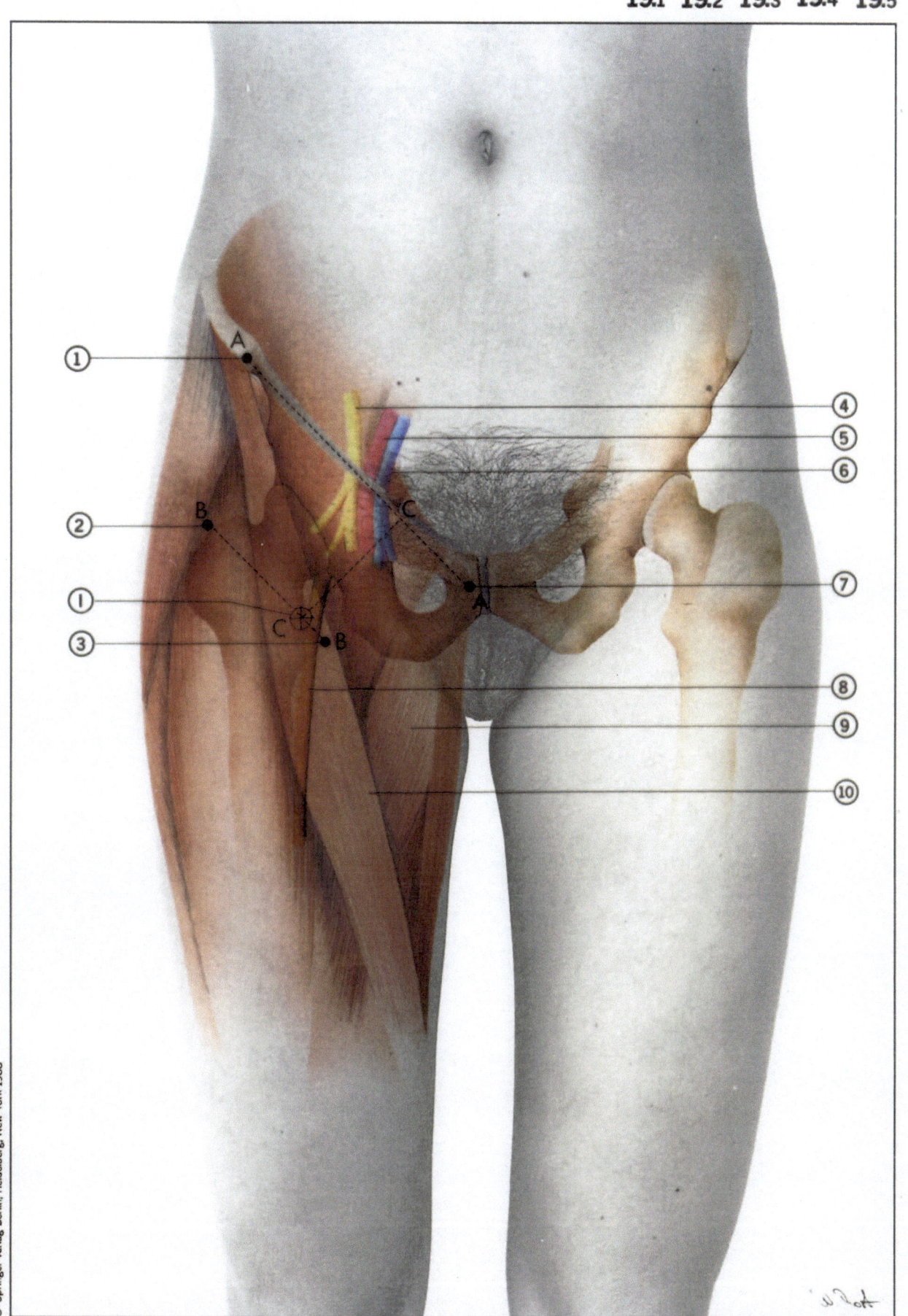

① Injection site for sciatic nerve block (supine anterior approach). A – – – – A: Line from anterior superior iliac spine to pubic tubercle.
B – – – – B: line from greater to lesser trochanter running parallel to line A – – A. C – – – – C: Line drawn perpendicular to A – – A and B – – B
at medial third of A – – A. ① Anterior superior iliac spine. ② Greater trochanter. ③ Lesser trochanter. ④ Femoral nerve. ⑤ Femoral artery.
⑥ Femoral vein. ⑦ Pubic tubercle. ⑧ Sciatic nerve. ⑨ Adductor longus muscle. ⑩ Sartorius muscle

① Injection site for sciatic nerve block (supine posterior approach). A – – – – A: Line joining greater trochanter and ischial tuberosity. ① Ischial tuberosity. ② Greater trochanter. ③ Sciatic nerve in the gluteal region. ④ Gluteus maximus muscle

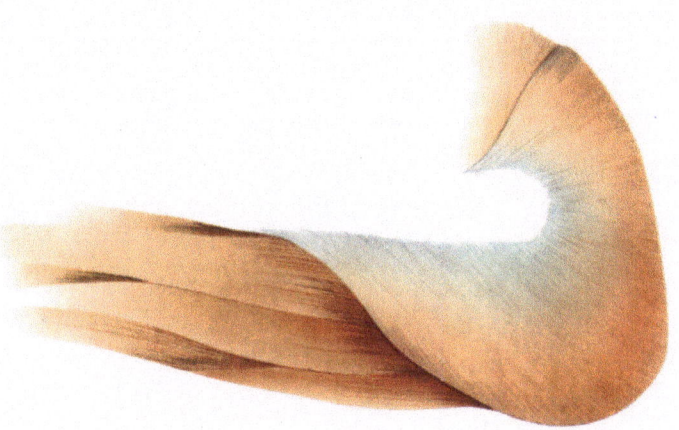

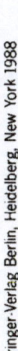

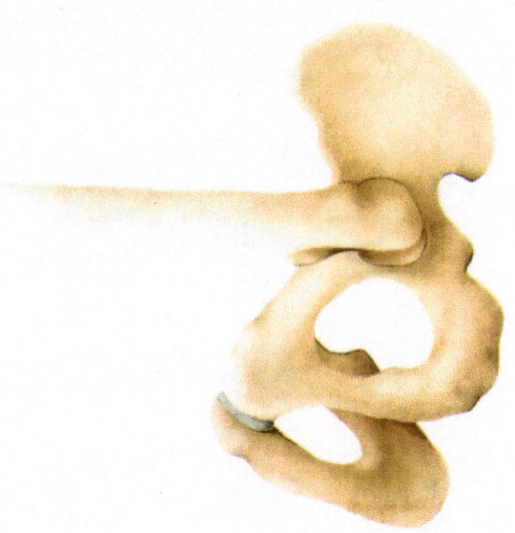

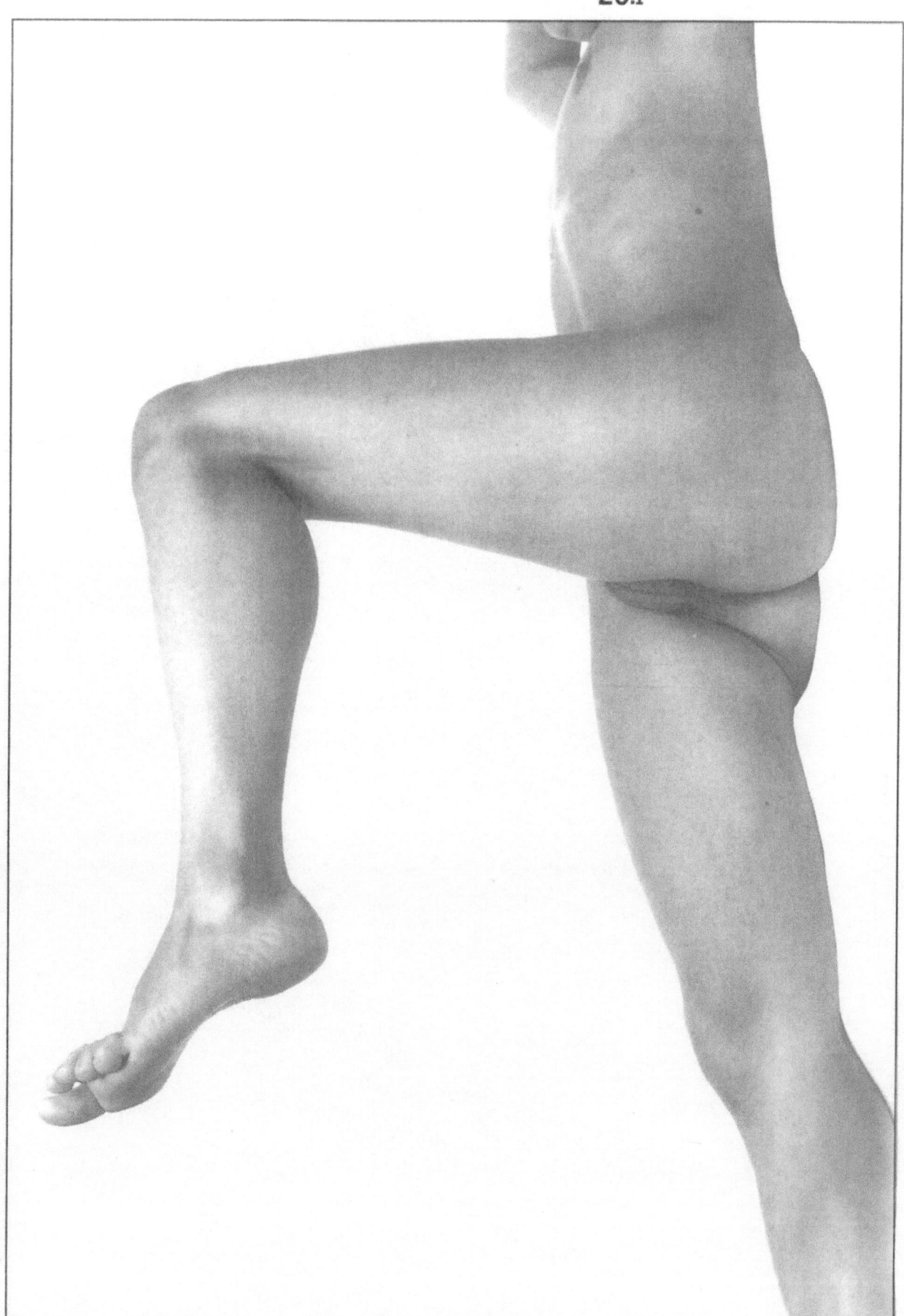

Sciatic Nerve Block: Supine Posterior Approach

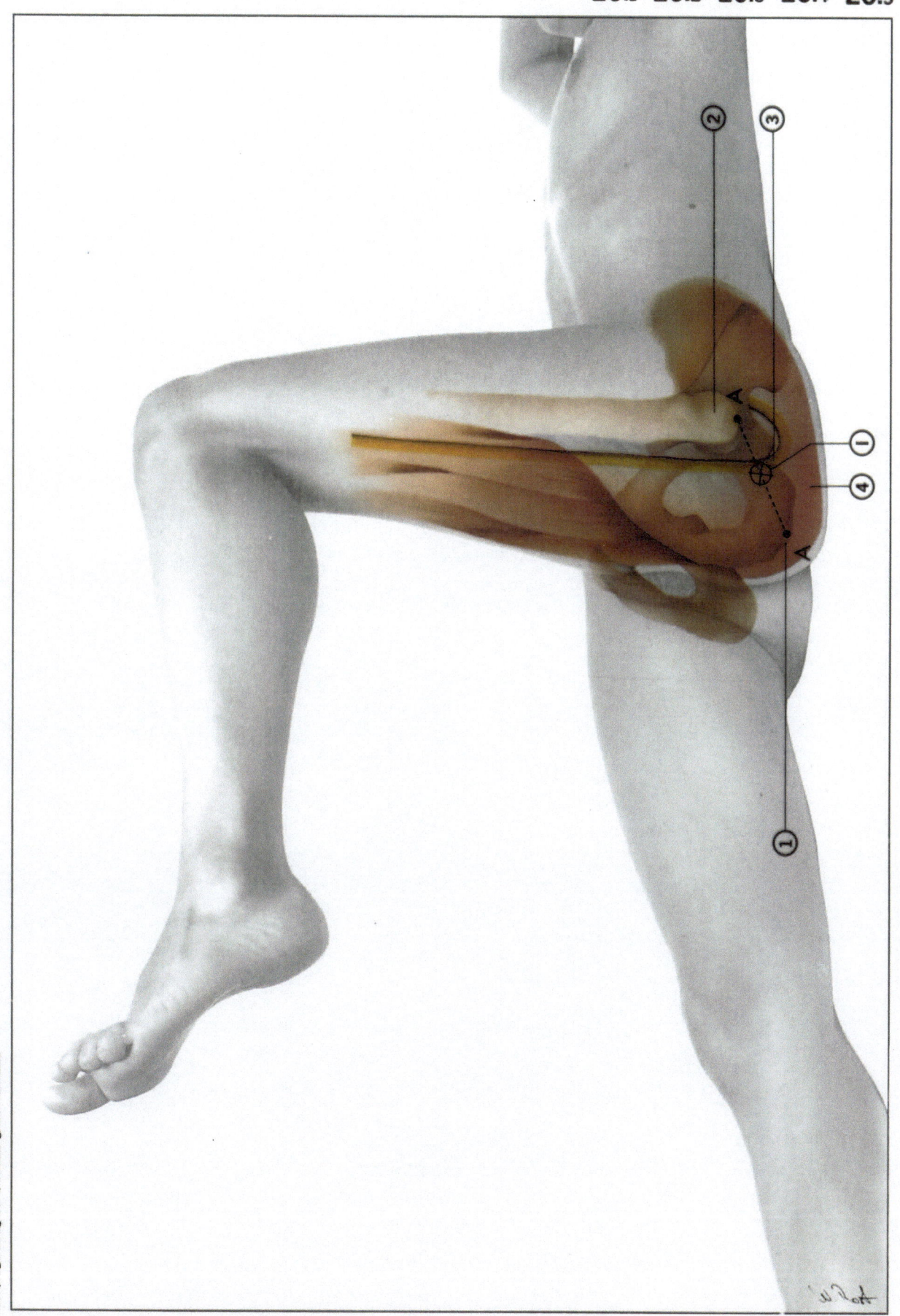

① Injection site for sciatic nerve block (supine posterior approach). A – – – – A: Line joining greater trochanter and ischial tuberosity. ① Ischial tuberosity. ② Greater trochanter. ③ Sciatic nerve in the gluteal region. ④ Gluteus maximus muscle

① Injection site for sciatic nerve block (supine lateral approach). A – – – – A: On the greater trochanter, a line is drawn across the posterior border extending caudad 1.5 – 2 cm from the superior border. ① Superior aspect of greater trochanter. ② Gluteus maximus muscle. ③ Sciatic nerve

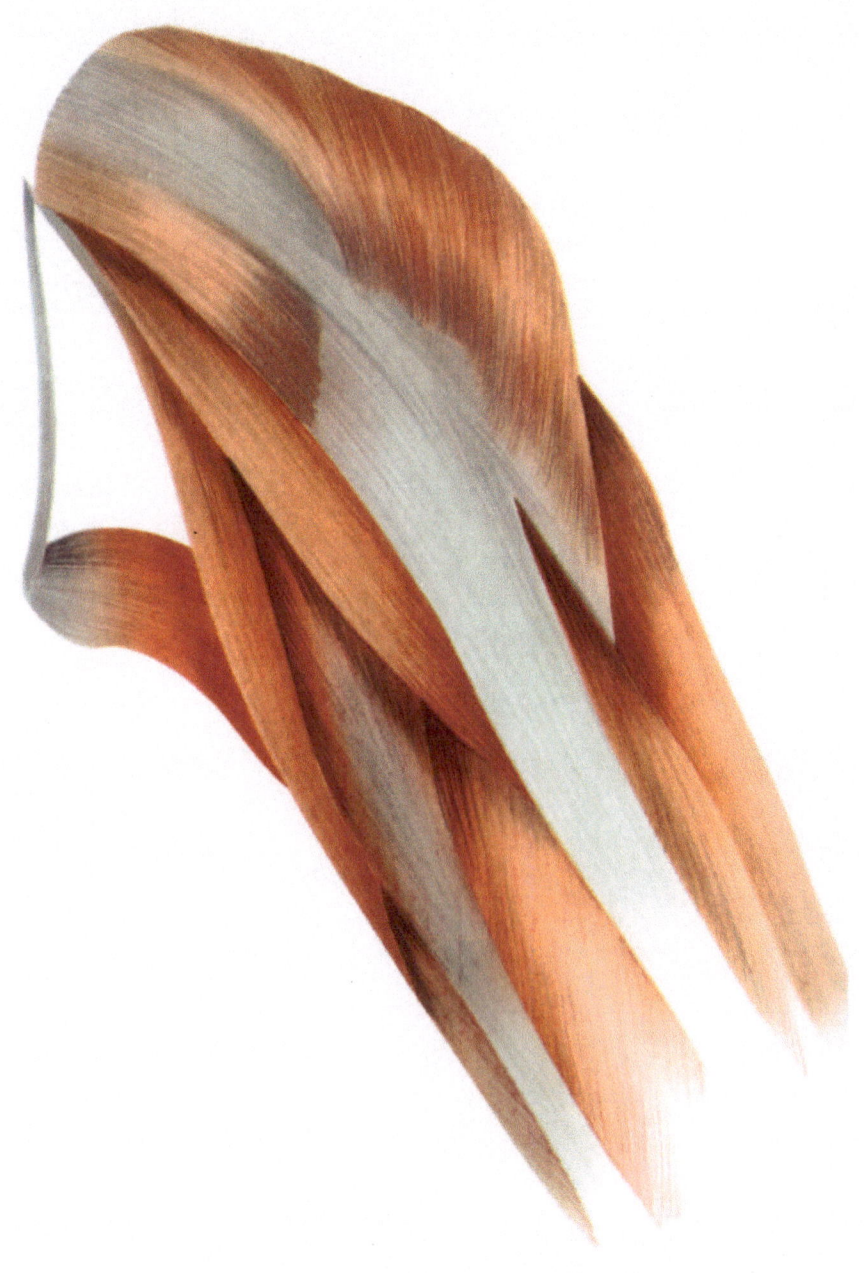

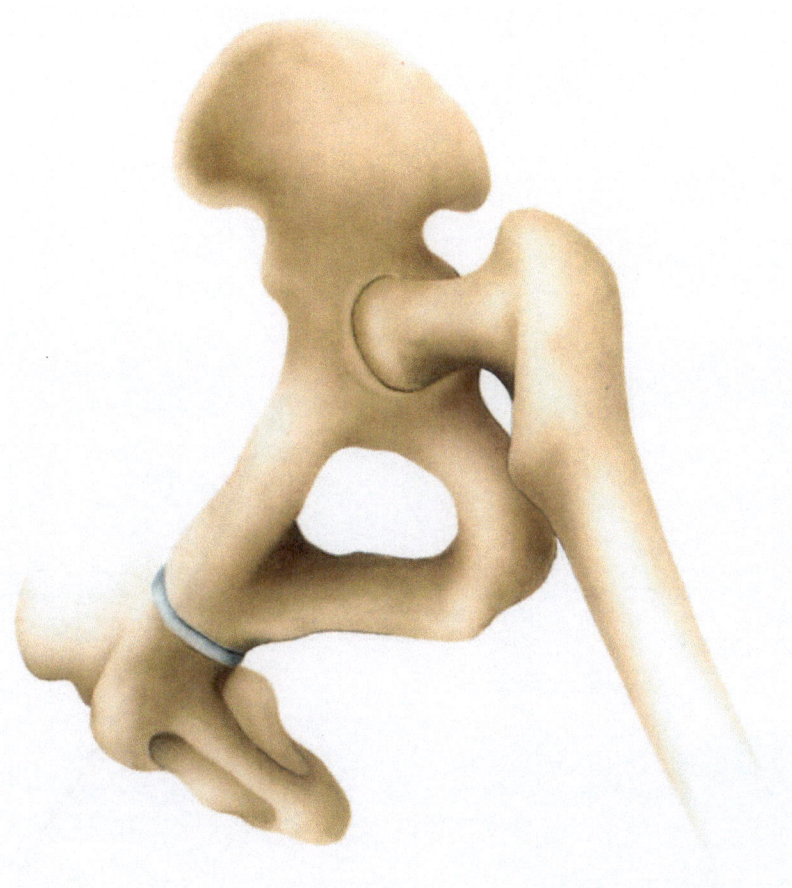

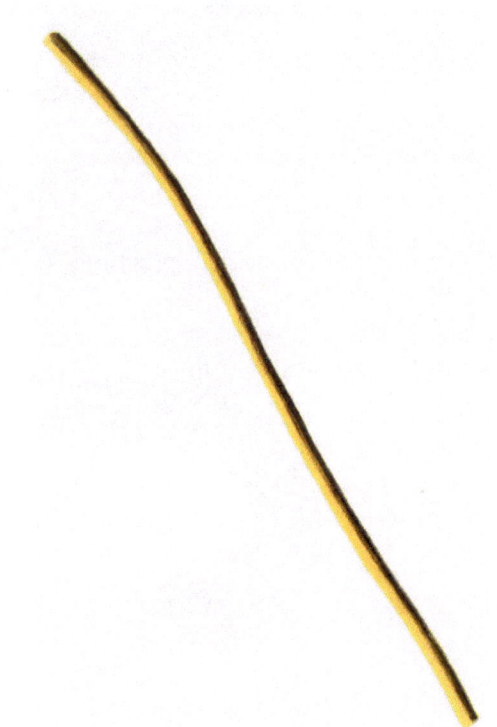

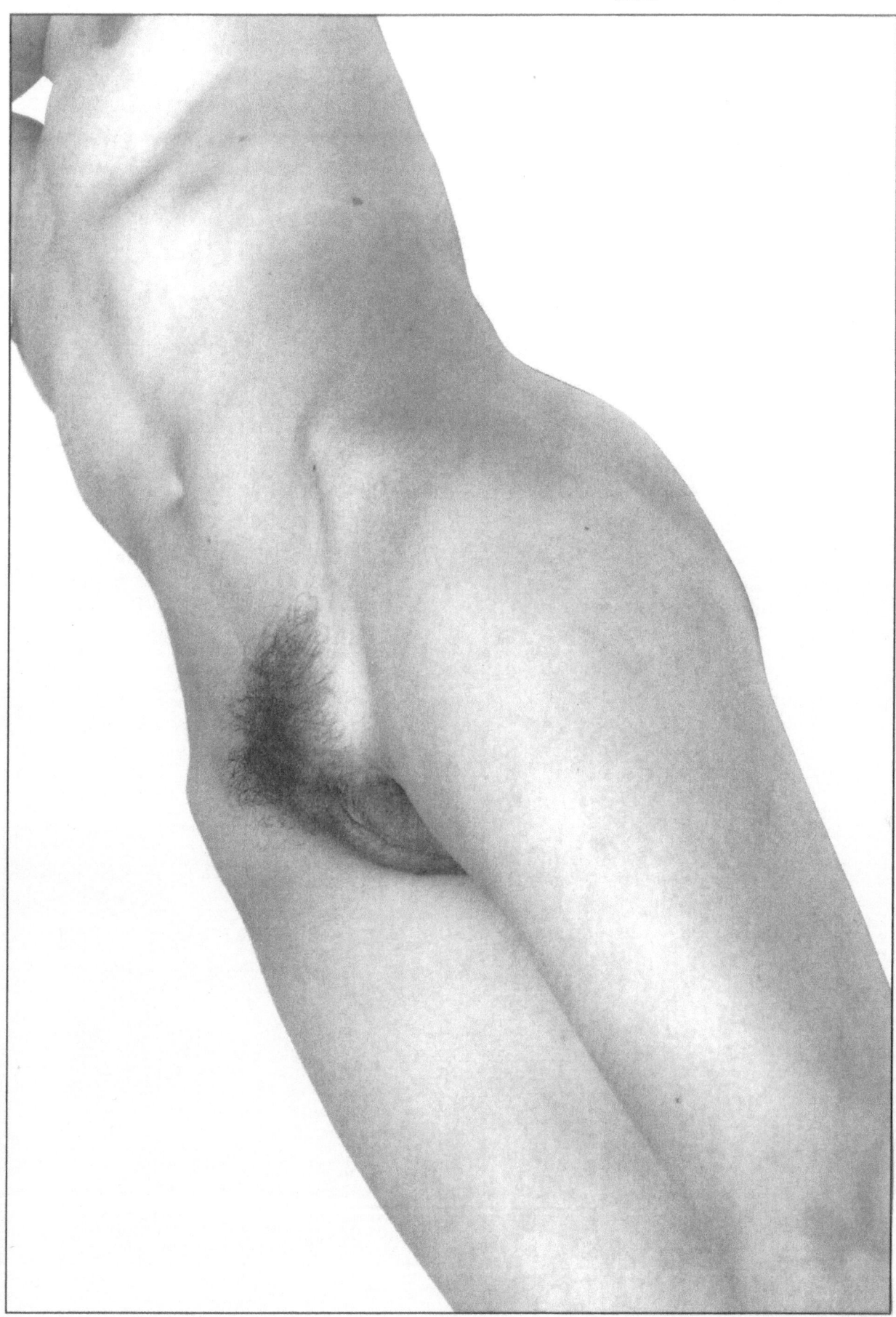

Sciatic Nerve Block: Supine Lateral Approach

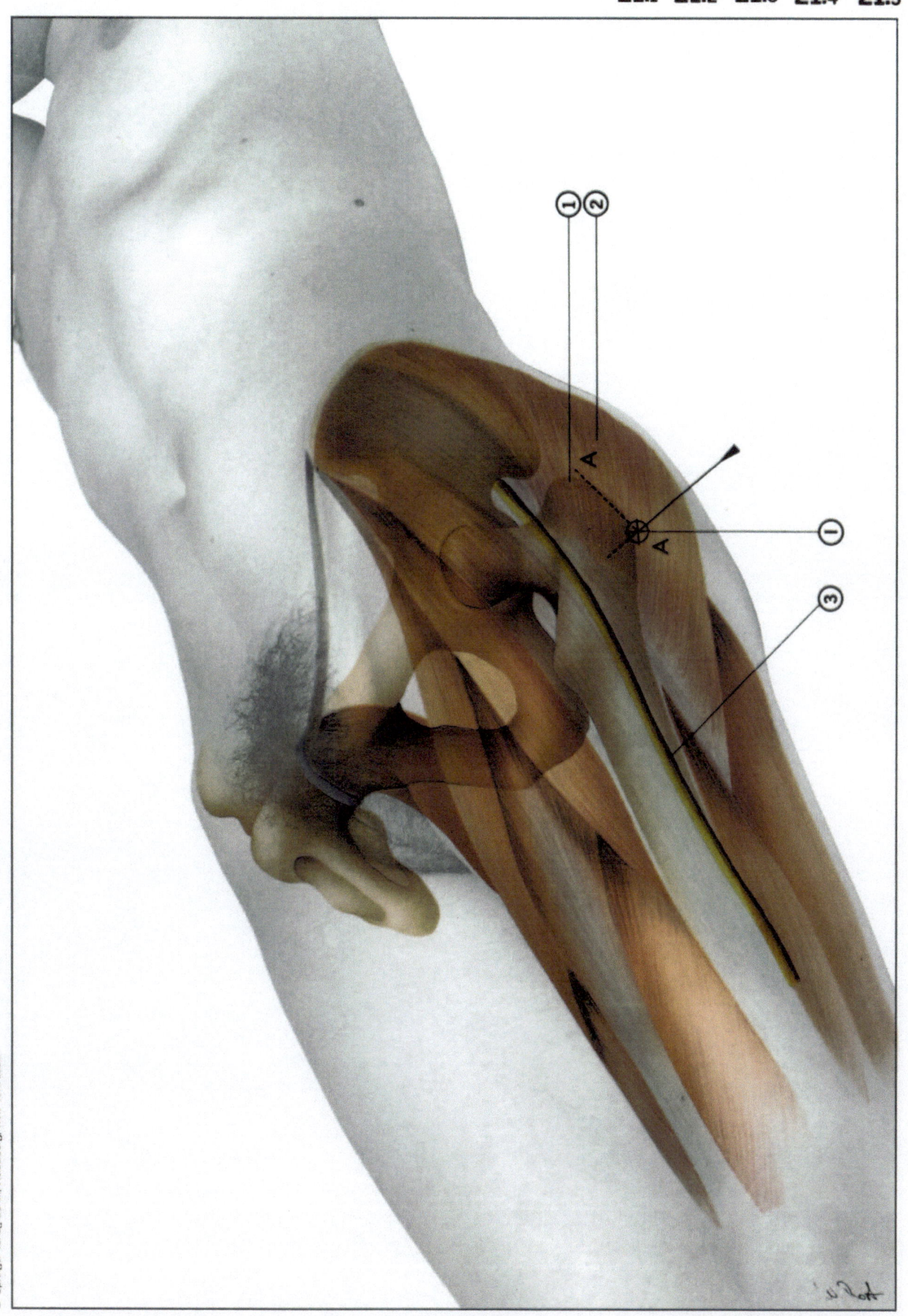

© Springer-Verlag Berlin, Heidelberg, New York 1988

① Injection site for sciatic nerve block (supine lateral approach). A – – – – A: On the greater trochanter, a line is drawn across the posterior border extending caudad 1.5 – 2 cm from the superior border. ① Superior aspect of greater trochanter. ② Gluteus maximus muscle. ③ Sciatic nerve

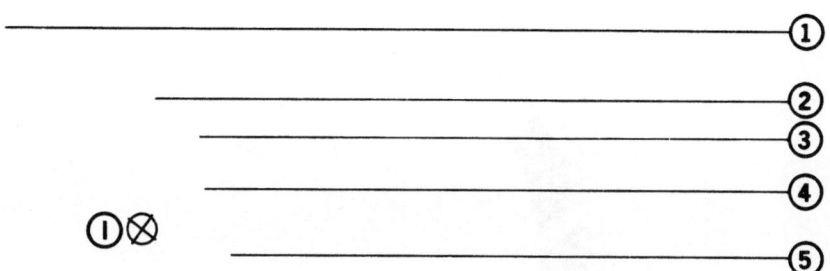

① Injection site for femoral nerve block. ① Anterior superior iliac spine. ② Femoral nerve. ③ Femoral artery. ④ Femoral vein. ⑤ Inguinal ligament

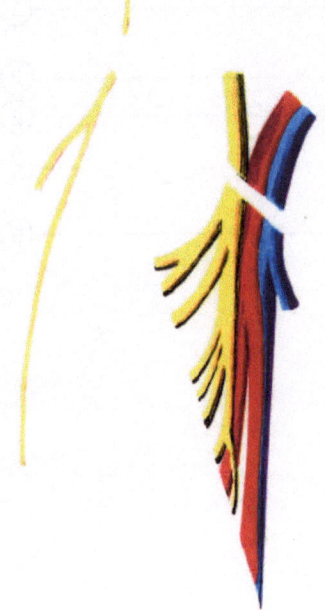

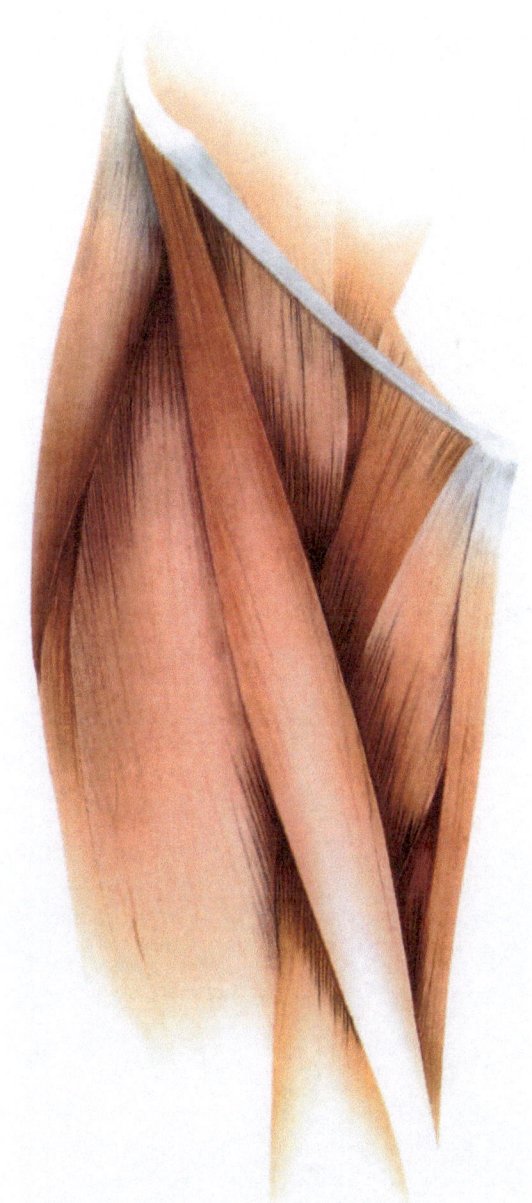

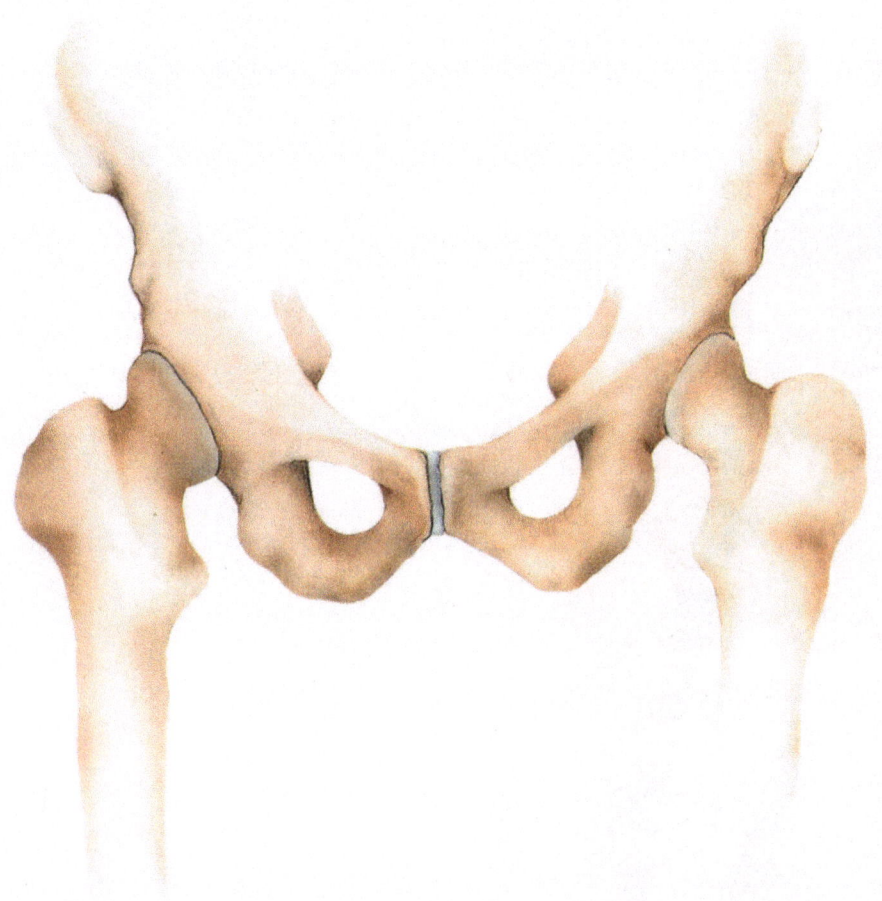

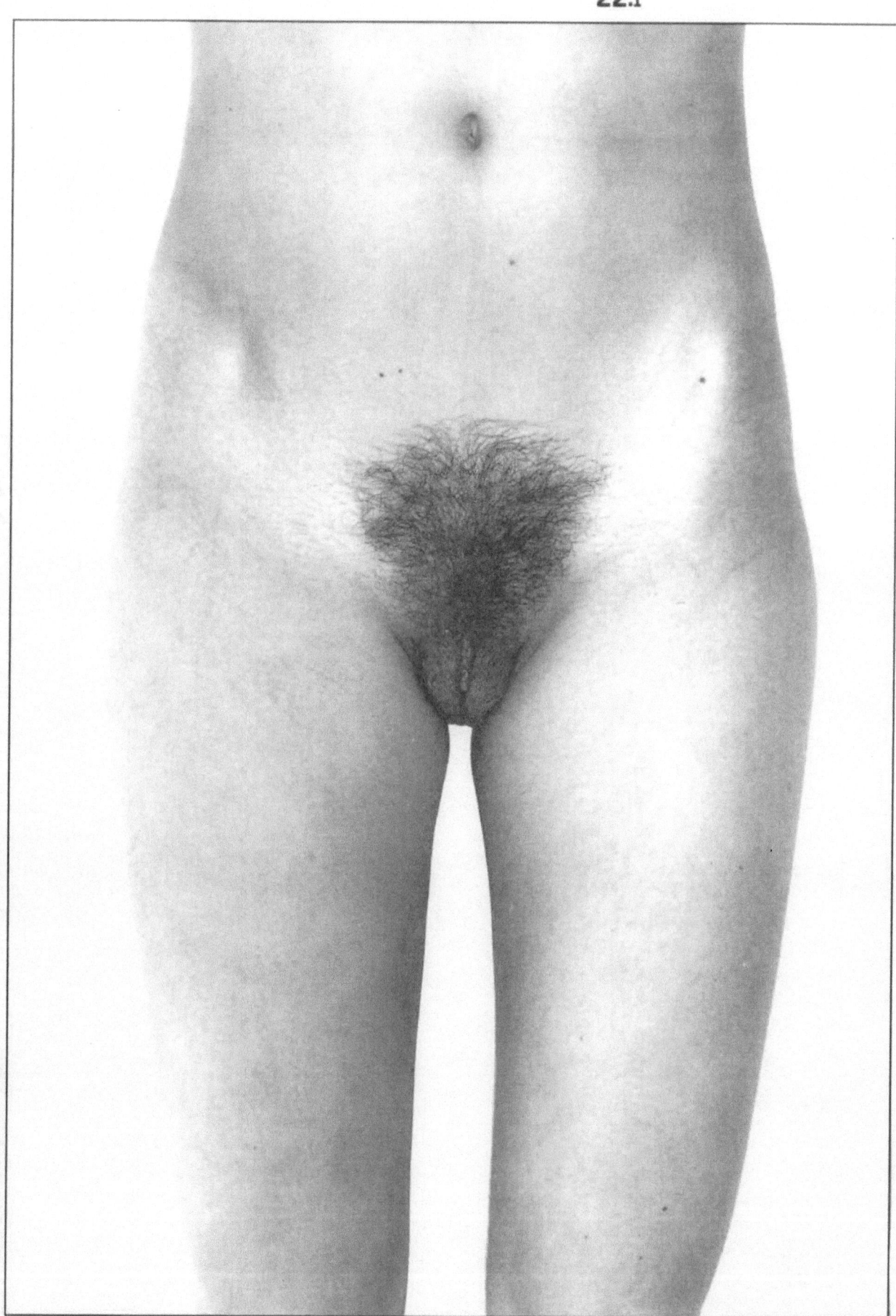

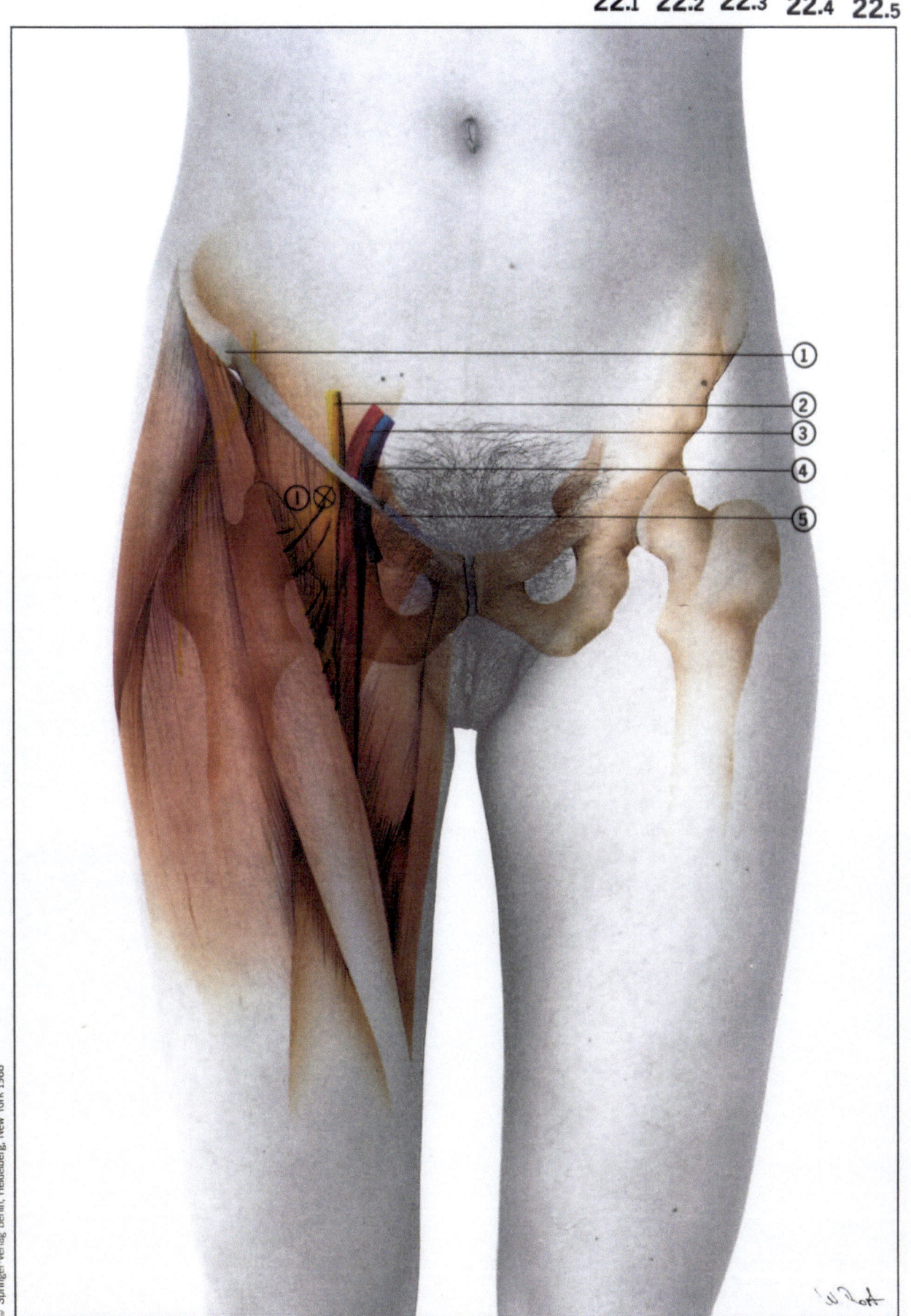

① Injection site for femoral nerve block. ① Anterior superior iliac spine. ② Femoral nerve. ③ Femoral artery. ④ Femoral vein. ⑤ Inguinal ligament

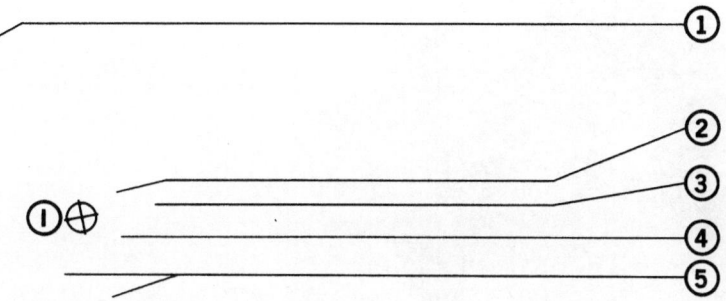

© Springer-Verlag Berlin, Heidelberg, New York 1988

① Injection site for obturator nerve block. ① Midpoint of inguinal ligament at which femoral artery can be palpated. ② Superior ramus of pubic bone. ③ Pubic tubercle. ④ Obturator foramen. ⑤ Anterior divisions of obturator nerve

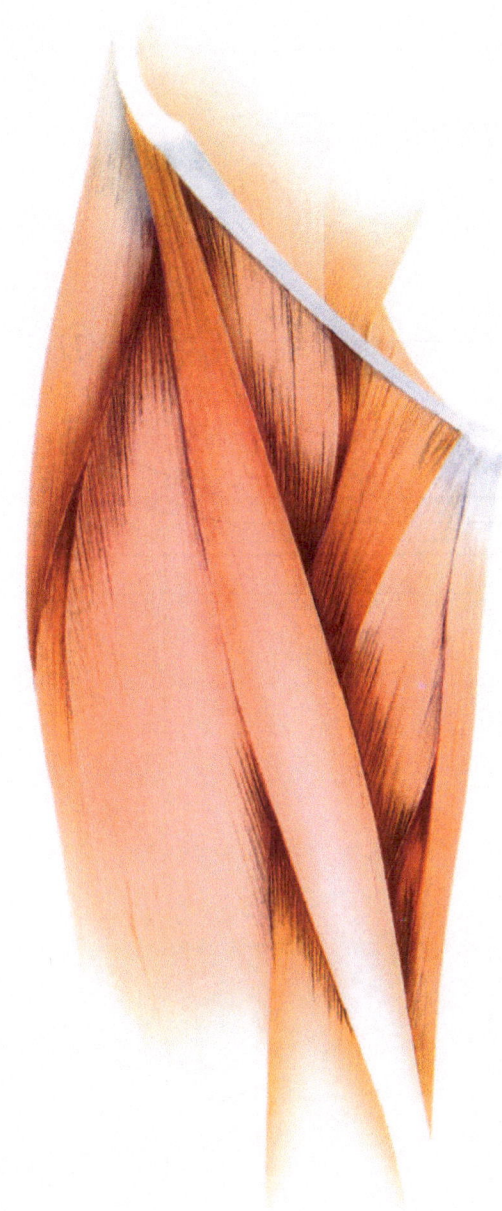

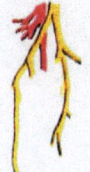

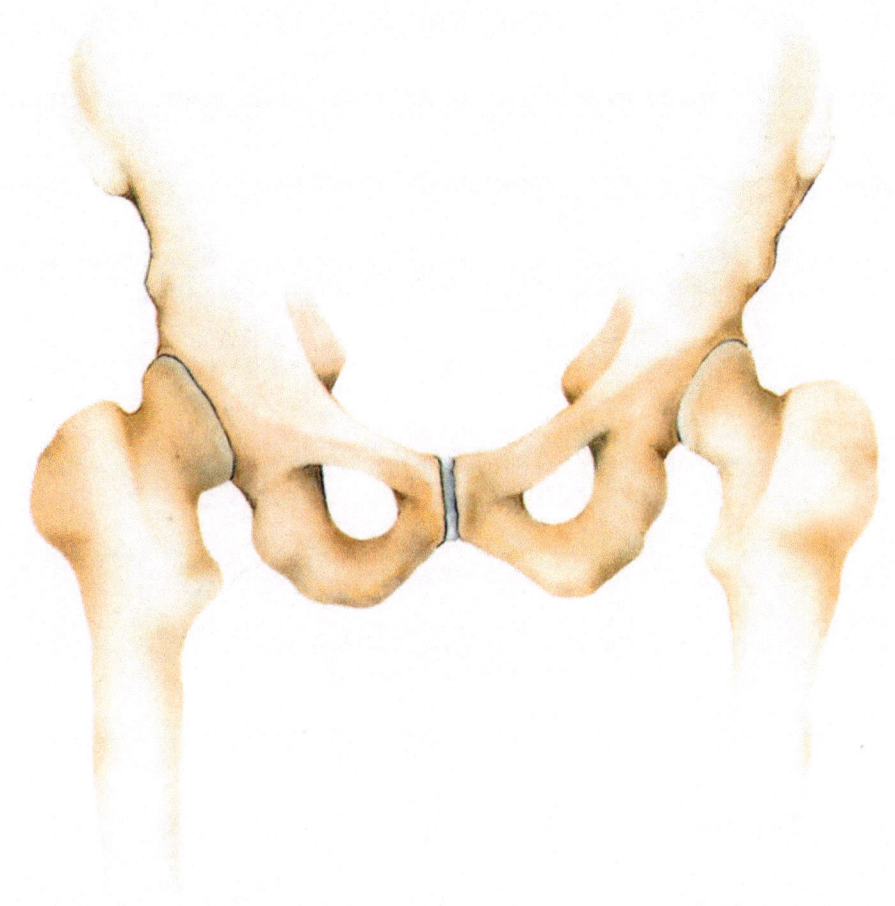

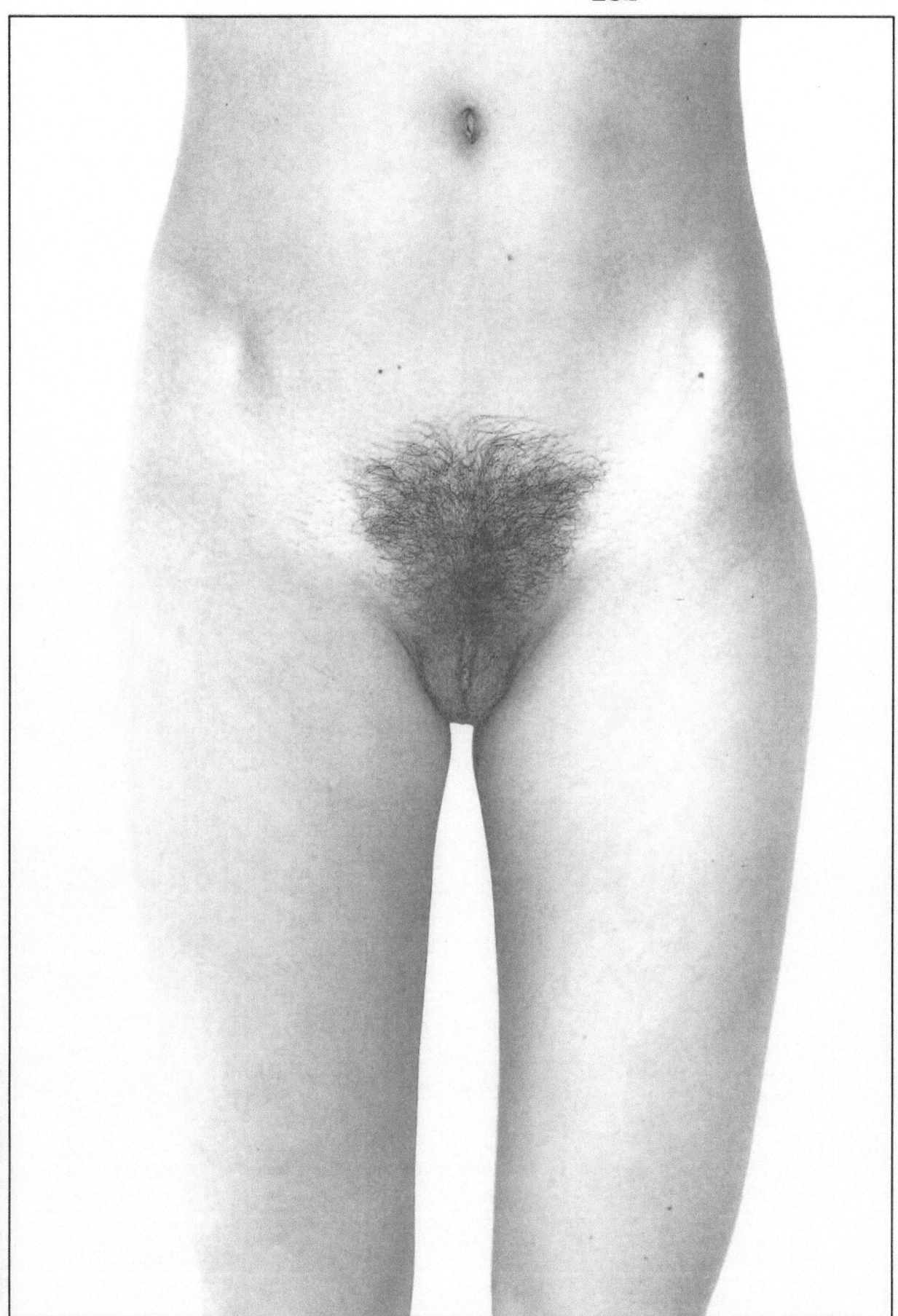

23

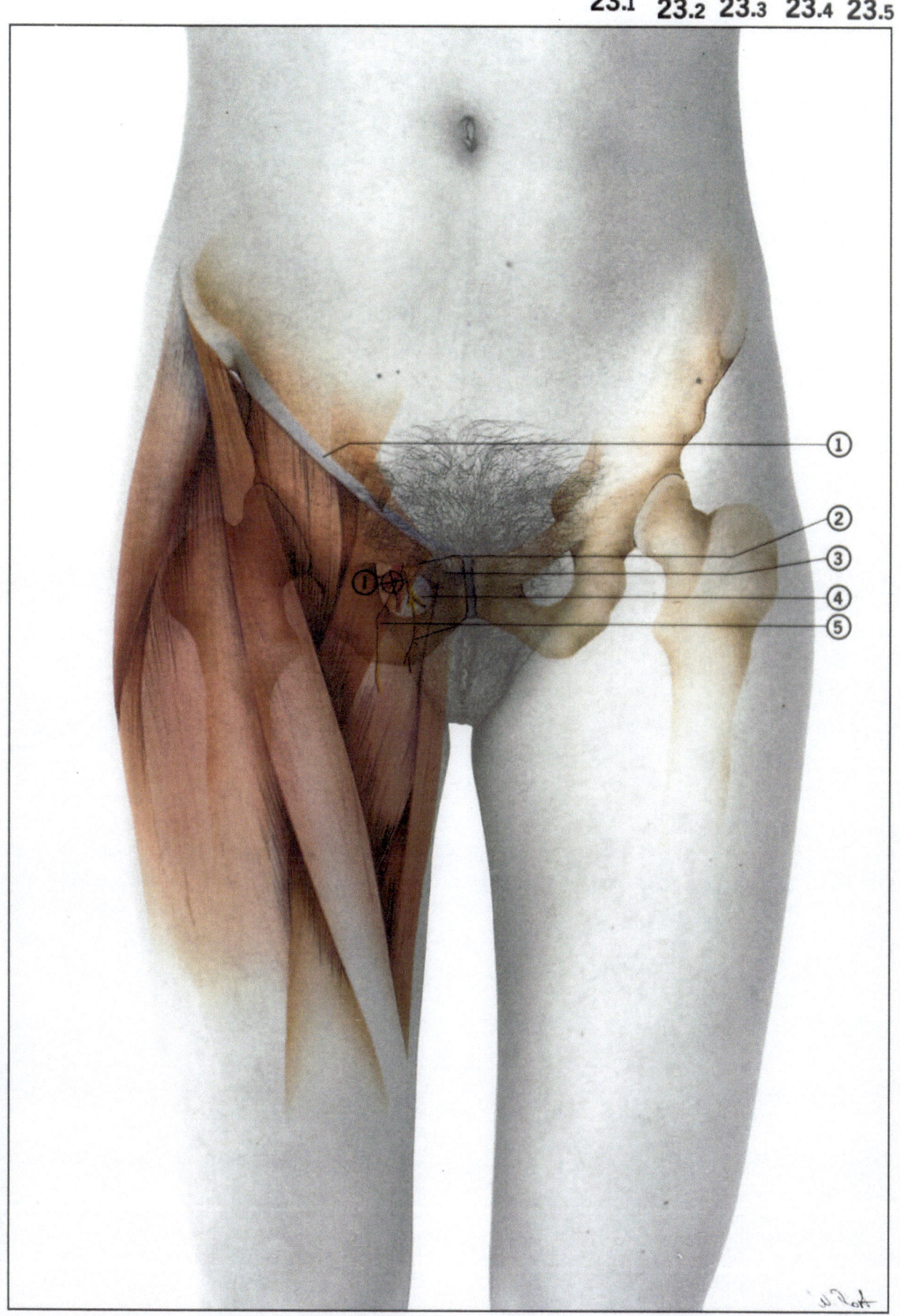

© Springer-Verlag, Berlin, Heidelberg, New York 1988

23

Injection site for obturator nerve block. ① Midpoint of inguinal ligament at which femoral artery can be palpated. ② Superior ramus of pubic bone. ③ Pubic tubercle. ④ Obturator foramen. ⑤ Anterior divisions of obturator nerve

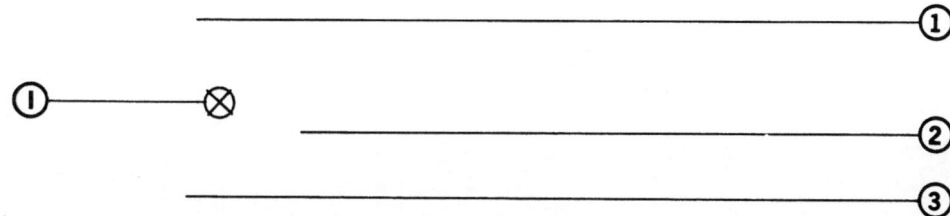

① Injection site for lateral femoral cutaneous nerve block. ① Anterior superior iliac spine. ② Inguinal ligament. ③ Lateral femoral cutaneous nerve

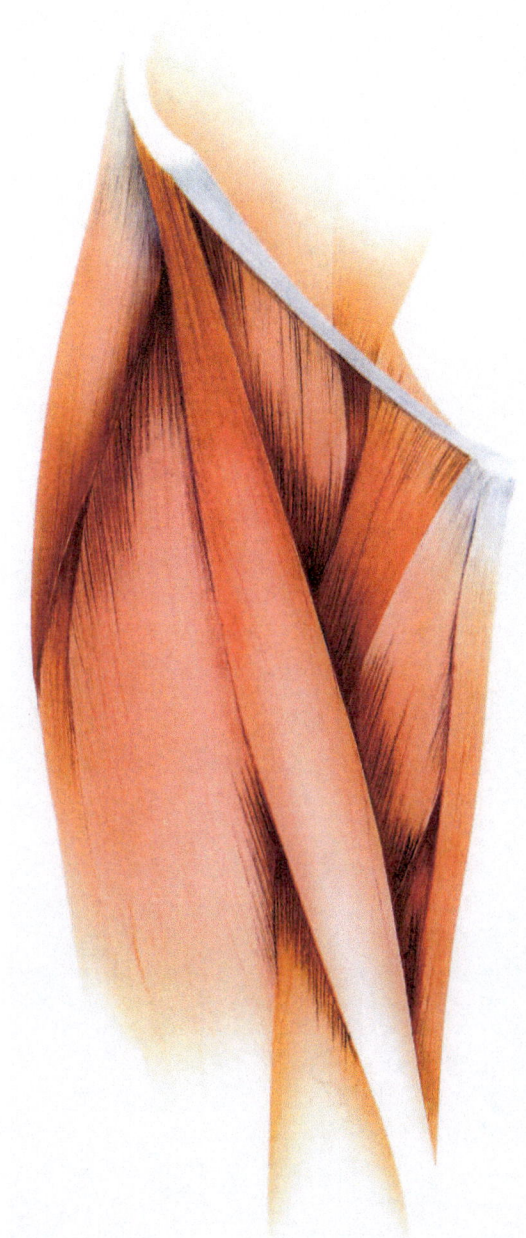

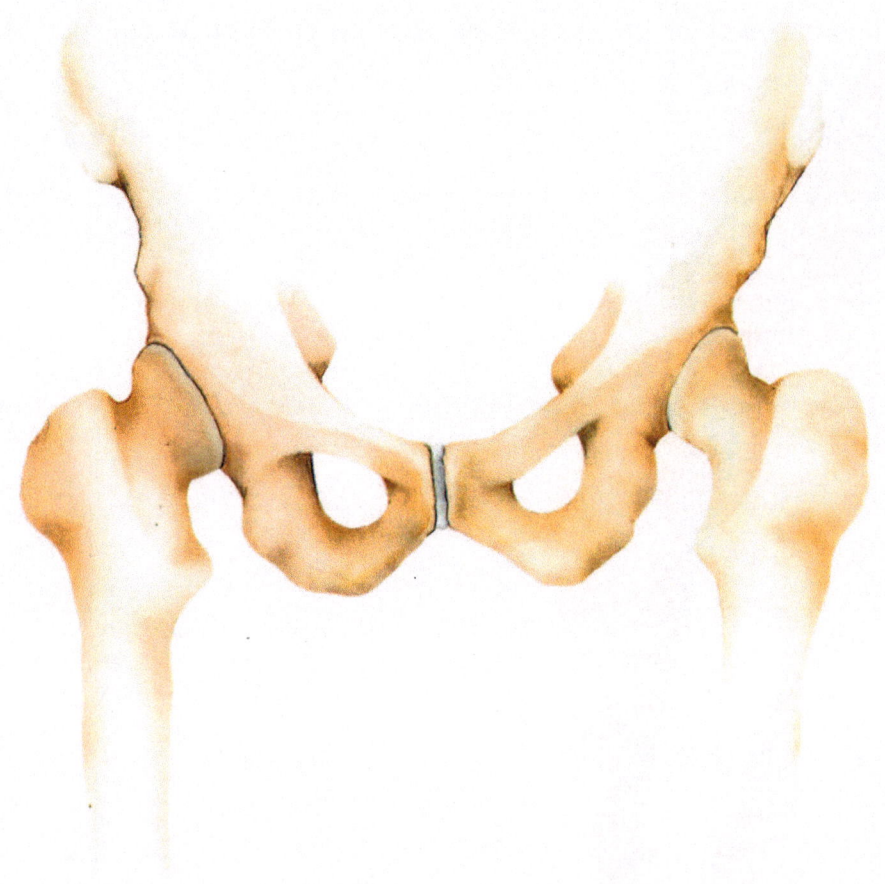

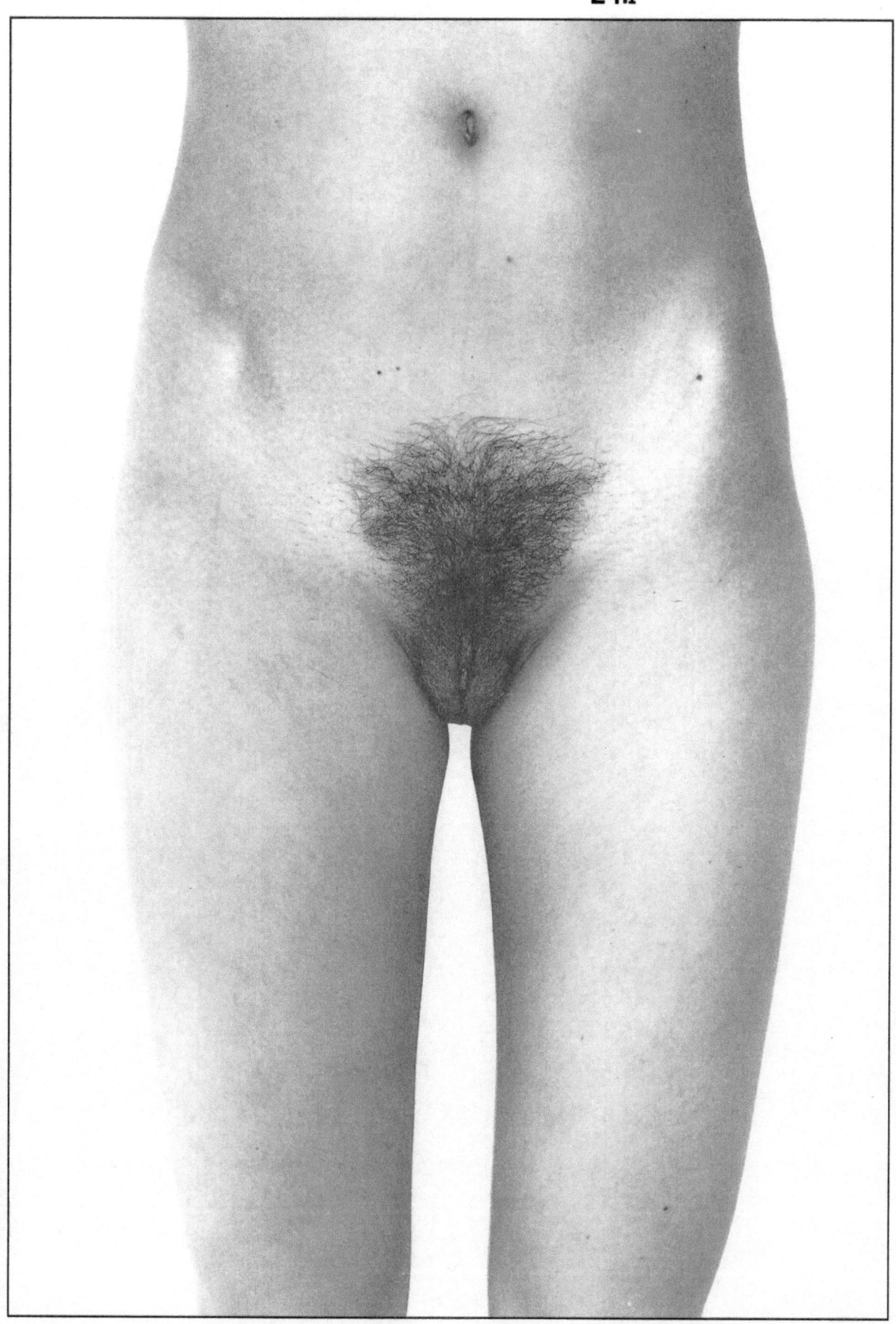

Lateral Femoral Cutaneous Nerve Block

Lateral Femoral Cutaneous Nerve Block

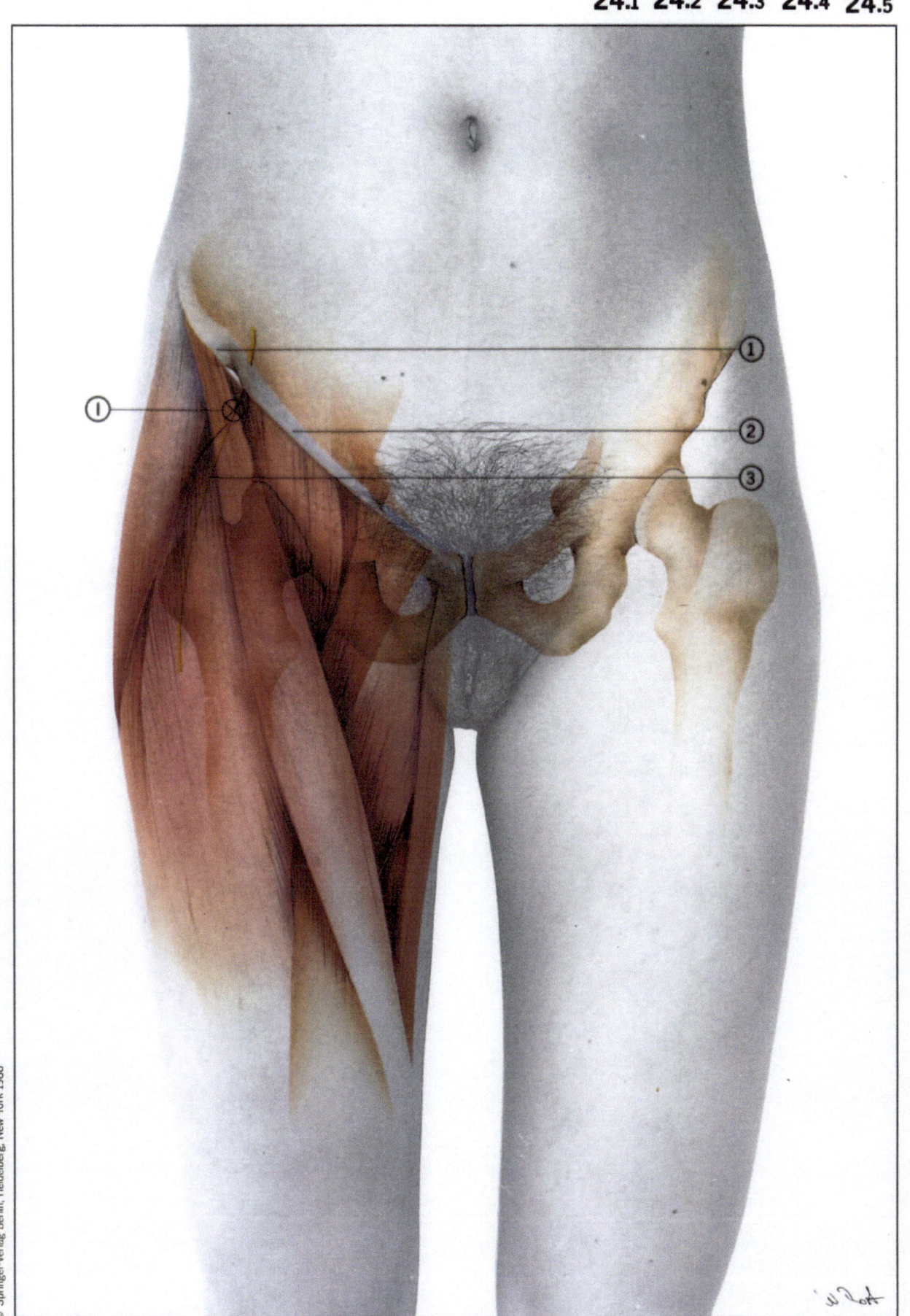

24

① Injection site for lateral femoral cutaneous nerve block. ① Anterior superior iliac spine. ② Inguinal ligament. ③ Lateral femoral cutaneous nerve

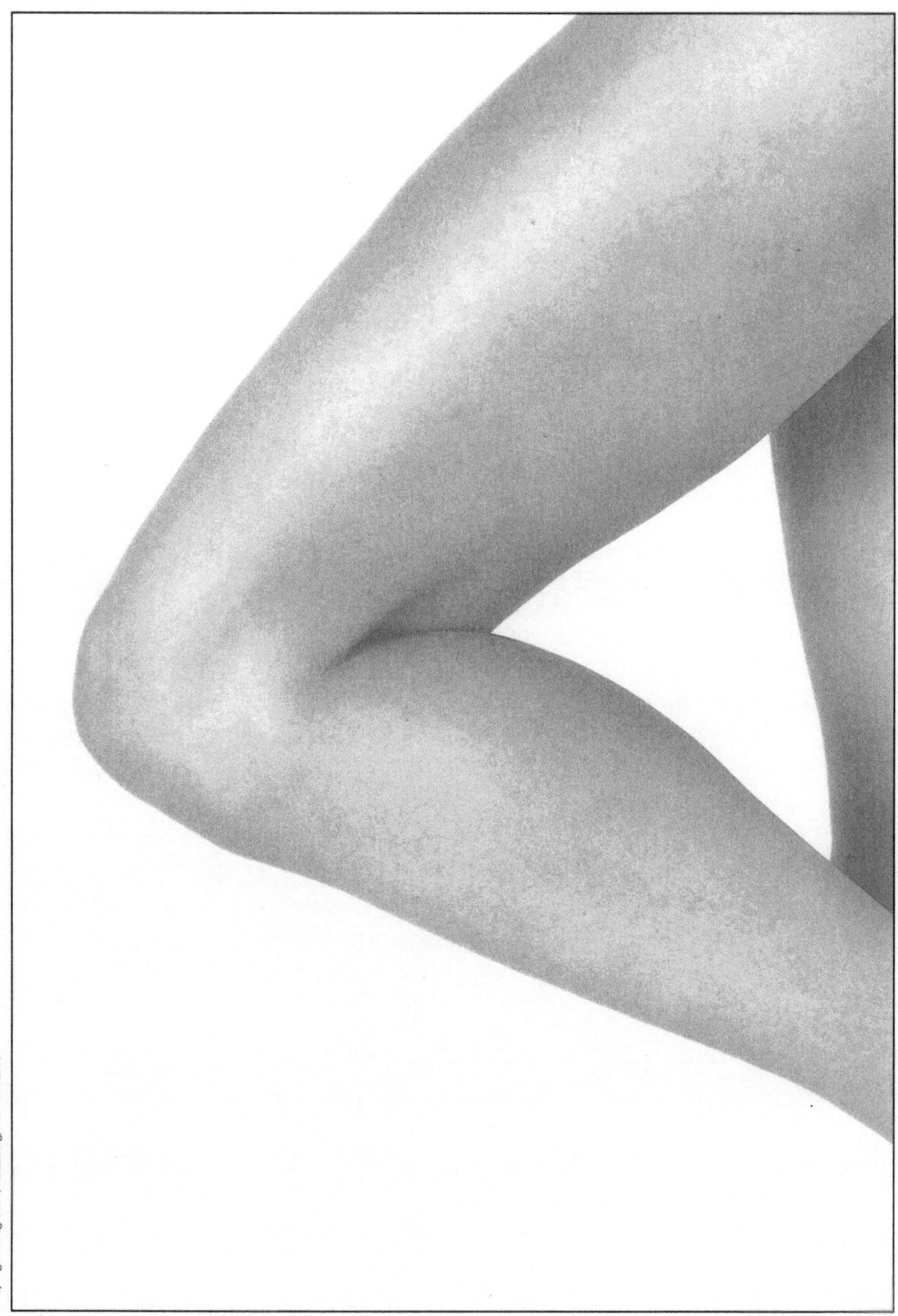

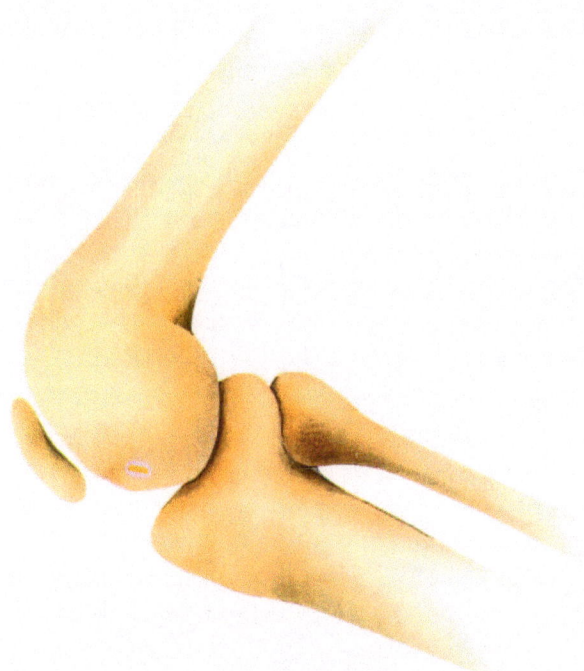

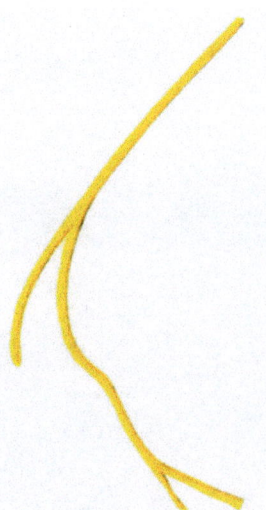

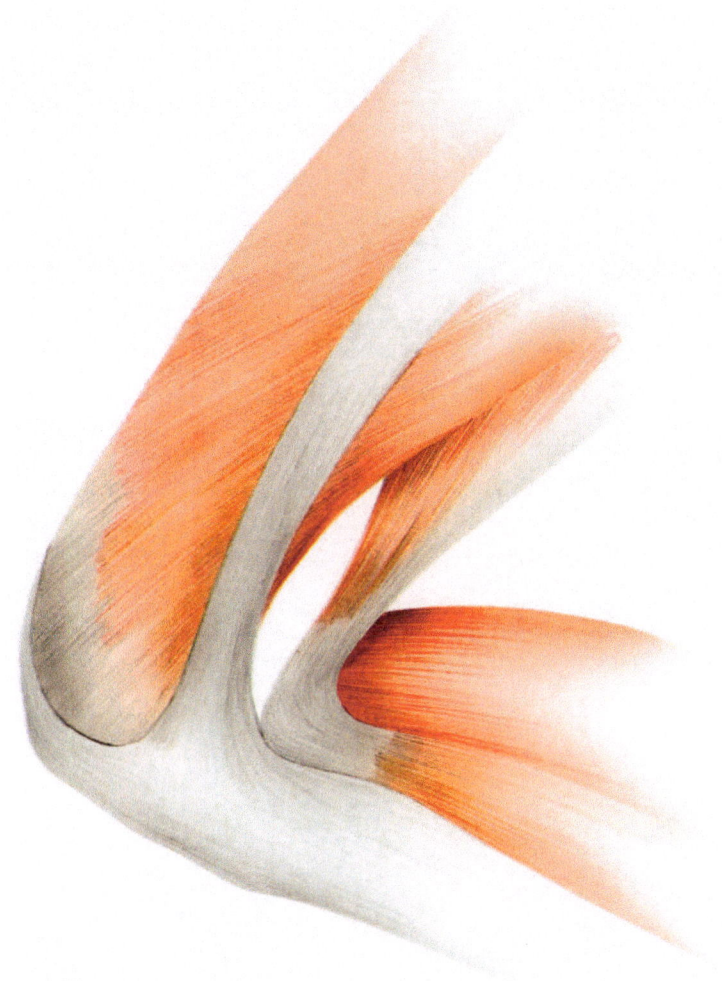

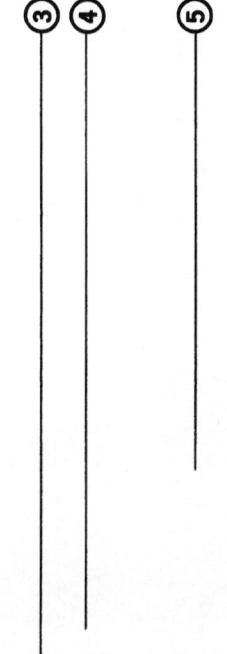

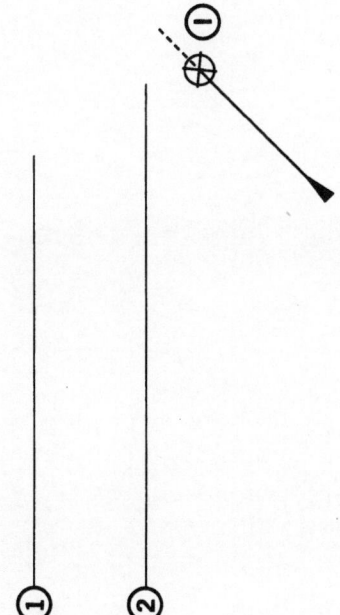

⊕ Injection site for common peroneal nerve block. ① Tibial plateau. ② Head of fibula. ③ Tibial nerve. ④ Common peroneal nerve. ⑤ Sciatic nerve

Common Peroneal and Tibial Nerve Block

25

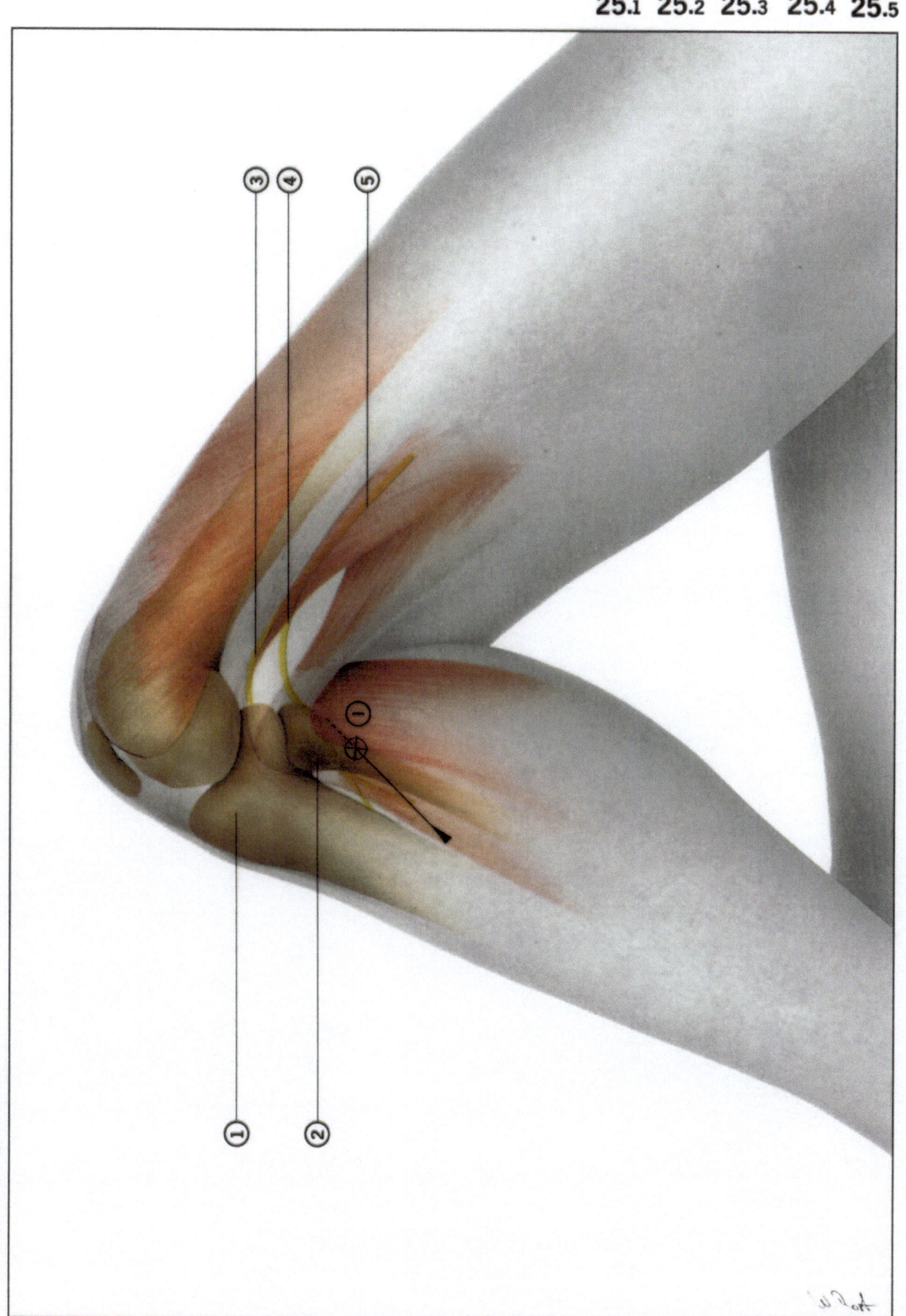

25

① Injection site for common peroneal nerve block. ① Tibial plateau. ② Head of fibula. ③ Tibial nerve. ④ Common peroneal nerve. ⑤ Sciatic nerve

① Injection site for saphenous nerve block. ① Patella. ② Medial condyle of femur. ③ Saphenous nerve. ④ Great saphenous vein. ⑤ Quadriceps femoris muscle

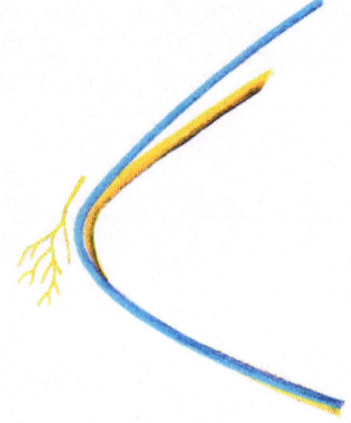

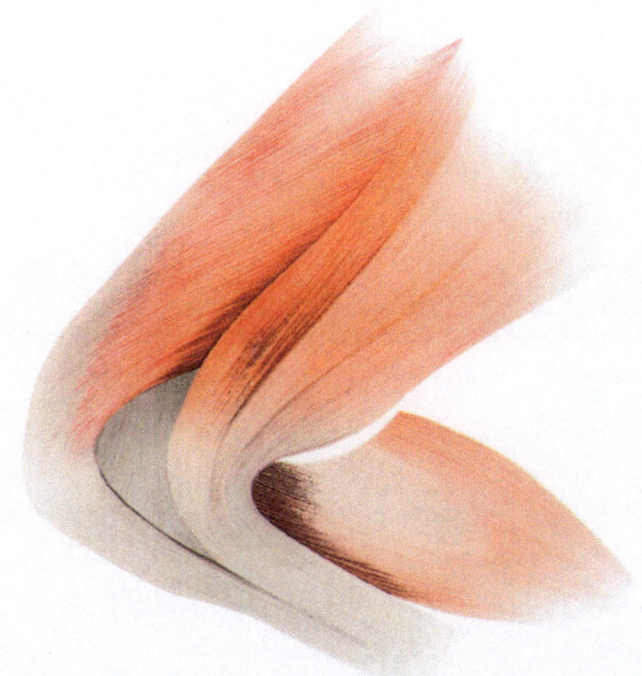

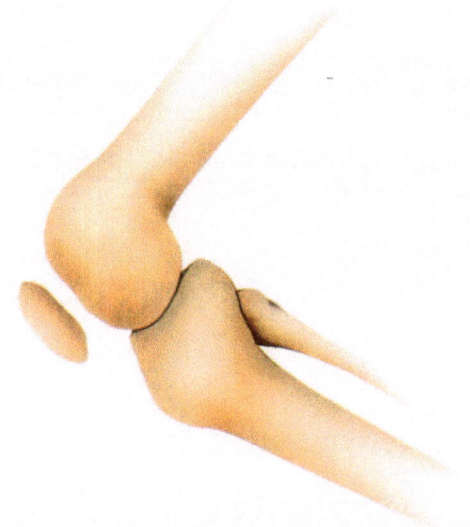

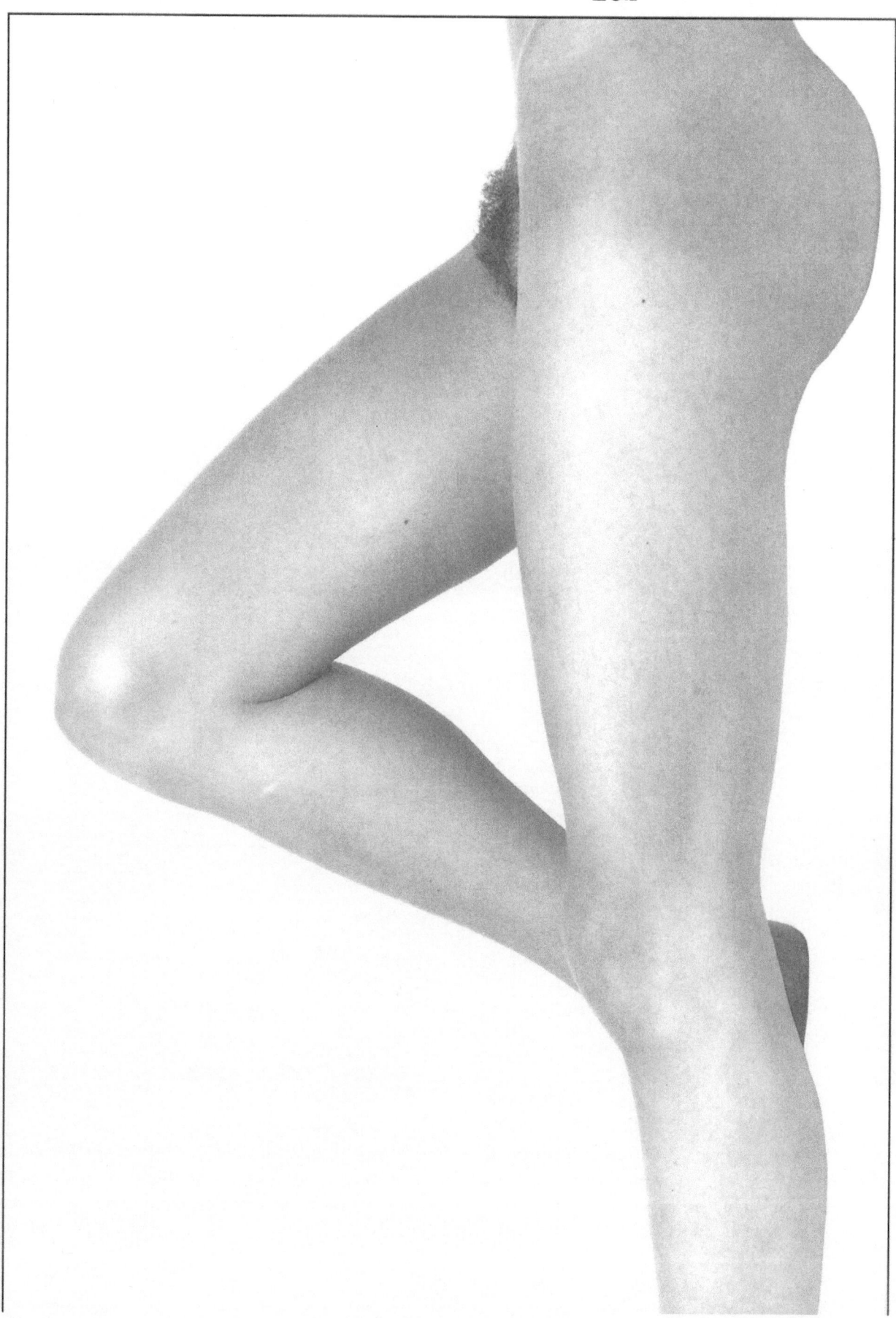

Saphenous Nerve Block at Knee

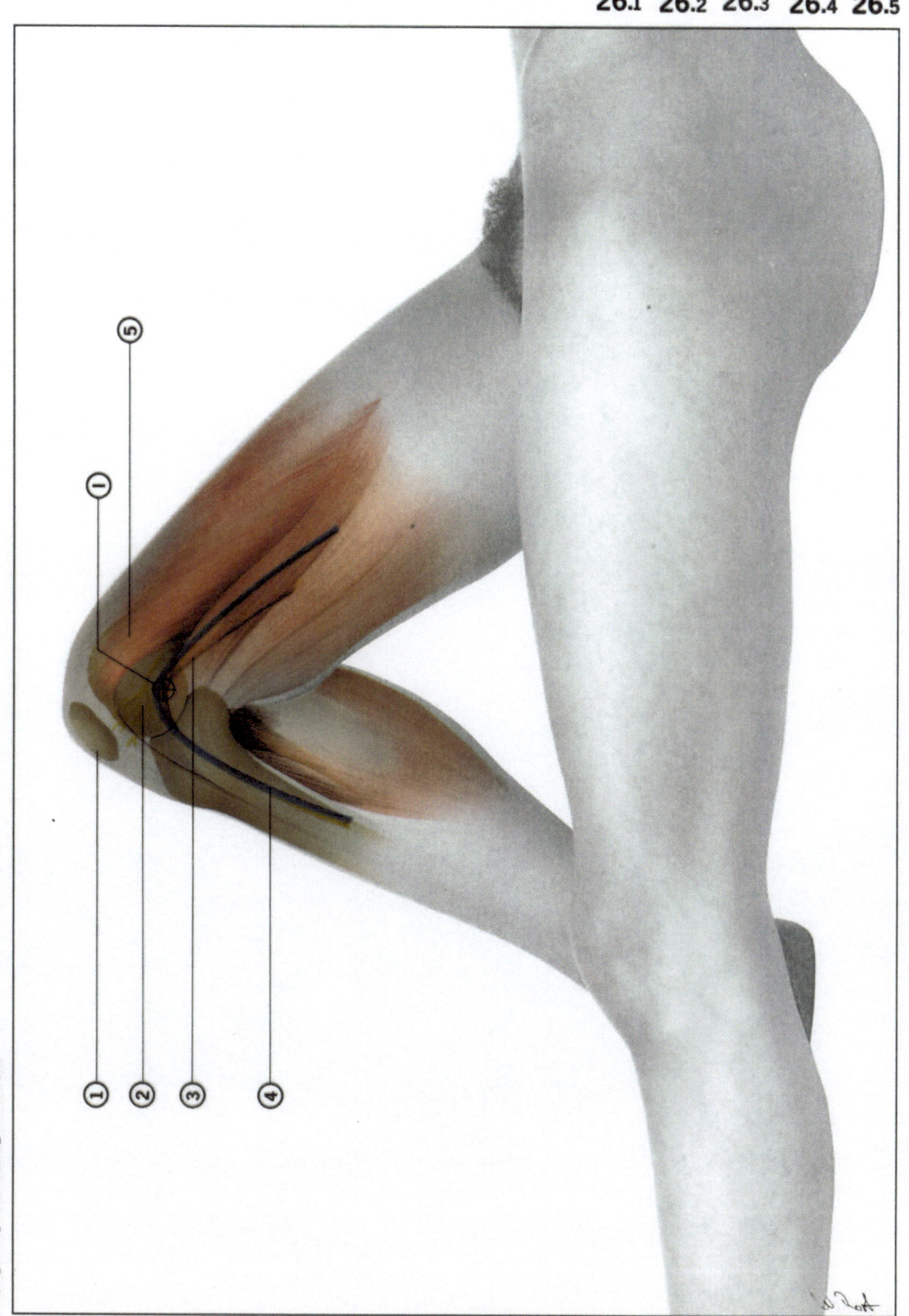

26

① Injection site for saphenous nerve block. ① Patella. ② Medial condyle of femur. ③ Saphenous nerve. ④ Great saphenous vein. ⑤ Quadriceps femoris muscle

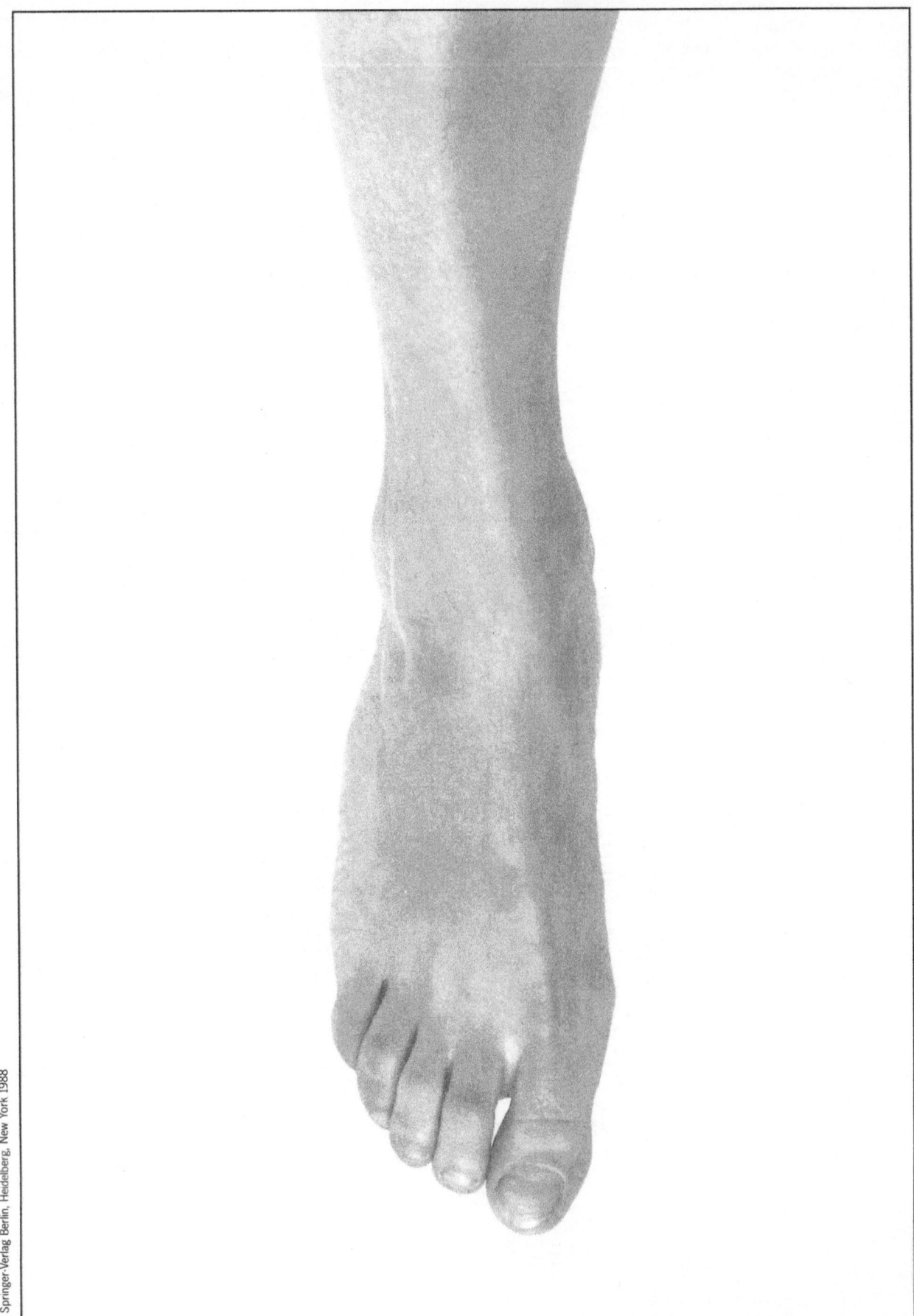

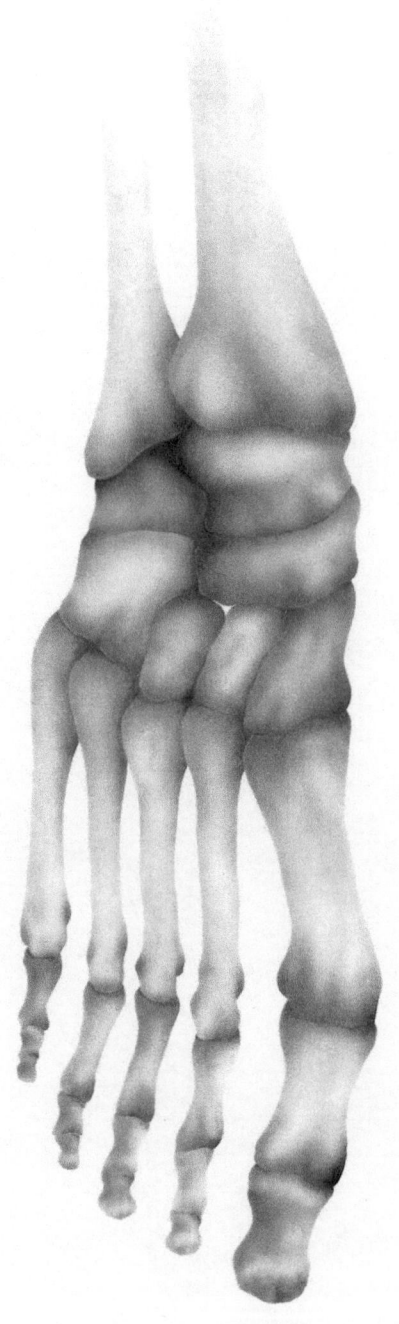

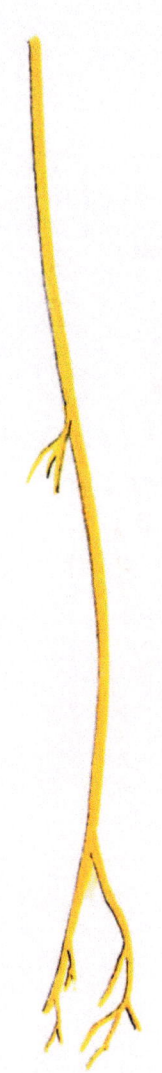

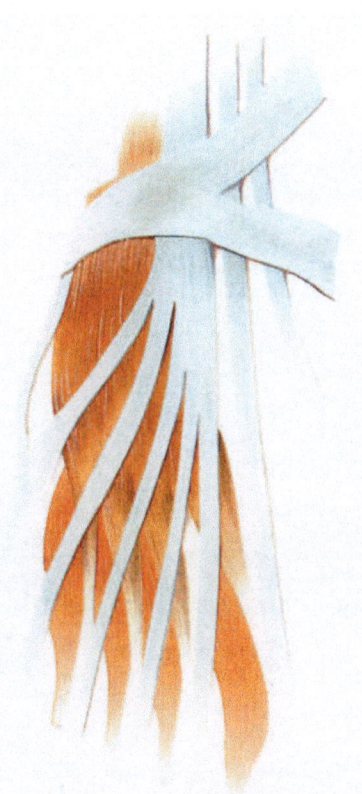

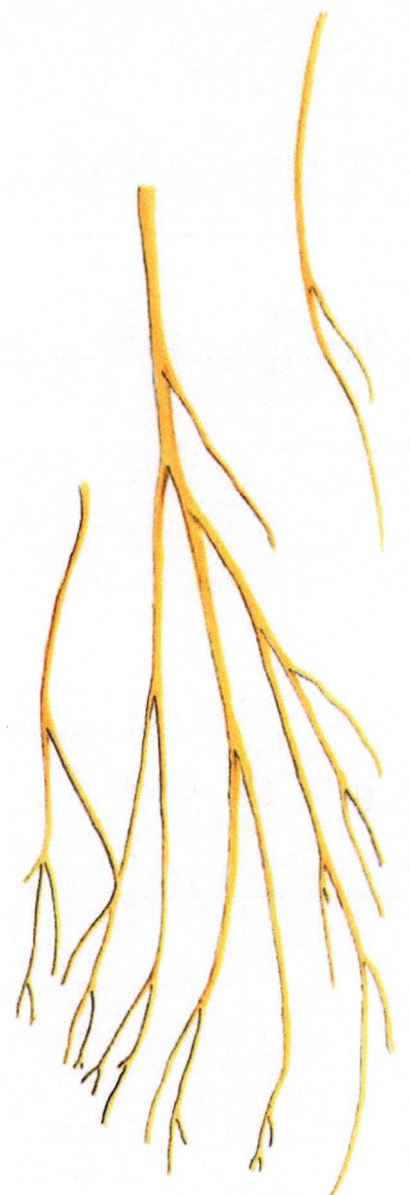

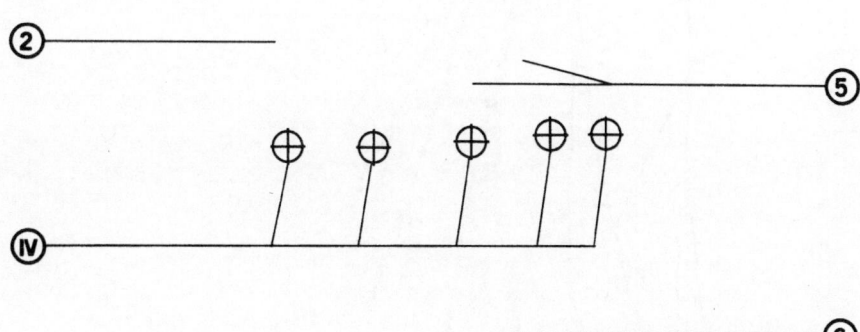

① Injection site for deep peroneal nerve block. ② Injection site for superficial peroneal nerve block. ③ Injection site for saphenous nerve block. ④ Injection sites for metatarsal nerve blocks. A – – – – A: Line along which skin infiltration is carried out. ① Superficial peroneal nerve. ② Sural nerve. ③ Deep peroneal nerve. ④ Saphenous nerve. ⑤ Medial and lateral terminal branches of peroneal nerve. ⑥ Dorsal digital nerves

Anterior Ankle and Metatarsal Block

Anterior Ankle and Metatarsal Block

27.1 27.2 27.3 27.4 27.5 27.6

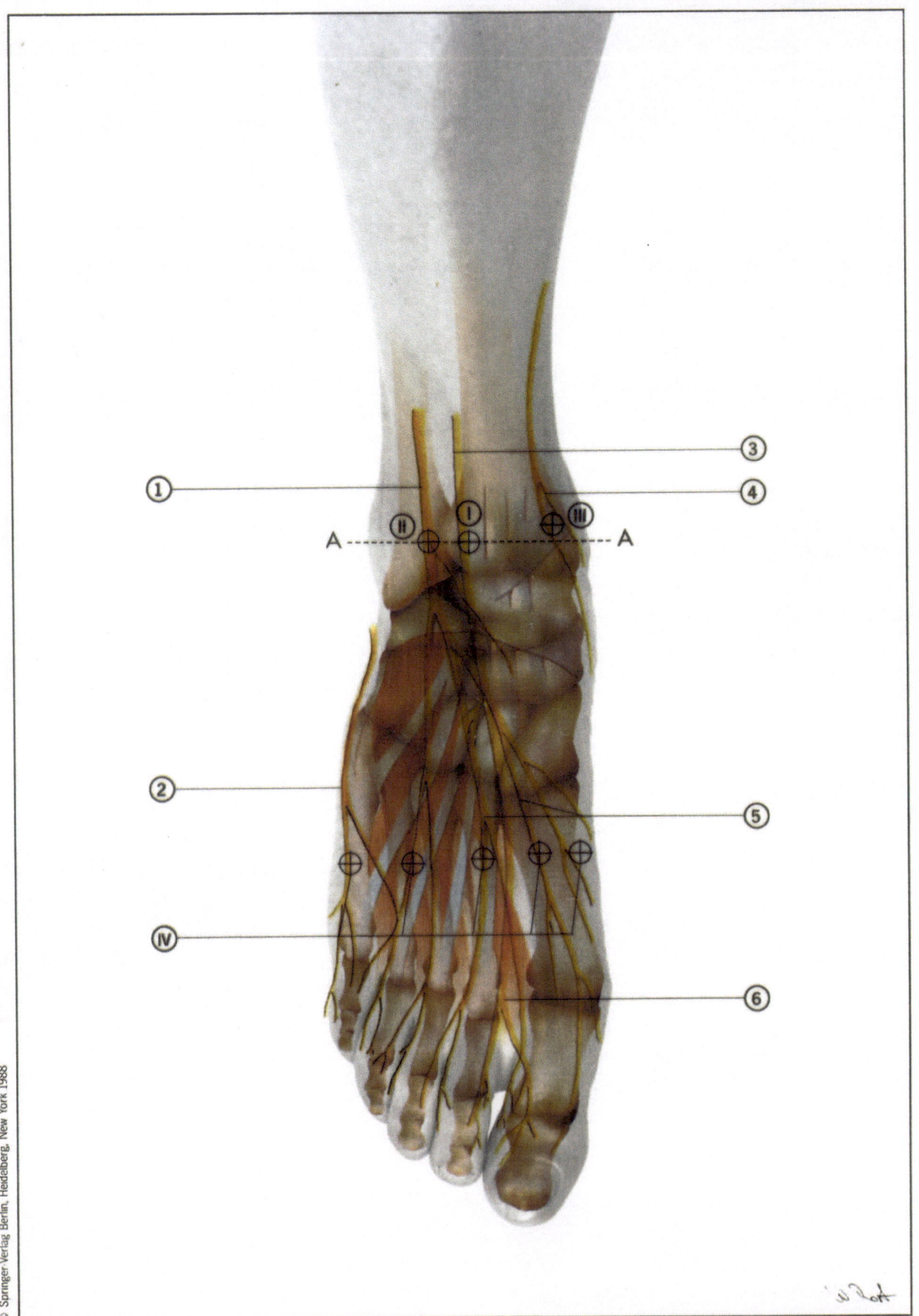

27

① Injection site for deep peroneal nerve block. ⑪ Injection site for superficial peroneal nerve block. ⑪⑪ Injection site for saphenous nerve block. ⑳ Injection sites for metatarsal nerve blocks. A – – – – A: Line along which skin infiltration is carried out. ① Superficial peroneal nerve. ② Sural nerve. ③ Deep peroneal nerve. ④ Saphenous nerve. ⑤ Medial and lateral terminal branches of peroneal nerve. ⑥ Dorsal digital nerves

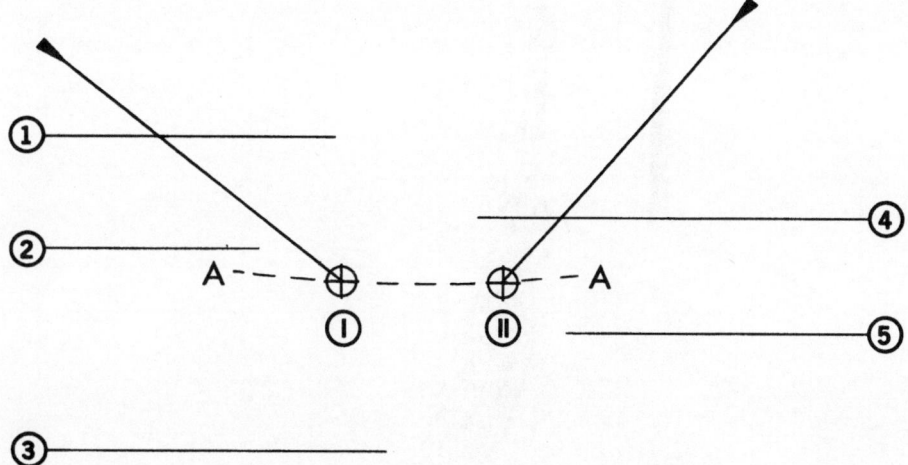

① Injection site for tibial nerve block at the ankle. ⑪ Injection site for sural nerve block at the ankle. A – – – – A: Line along which skin infiltration is carried out. ① Tibial nerve (alongside posterior tibial artery). ② Medial malleolus. ③ Flexor retinaculum ④ Sural nerve. ⑤ Lateral malleolus

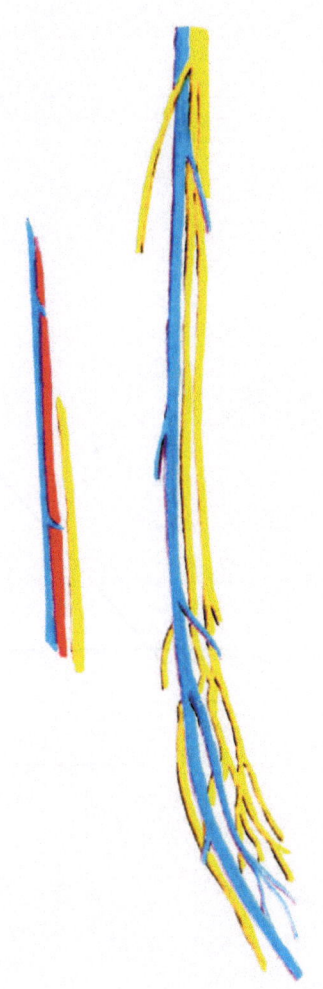

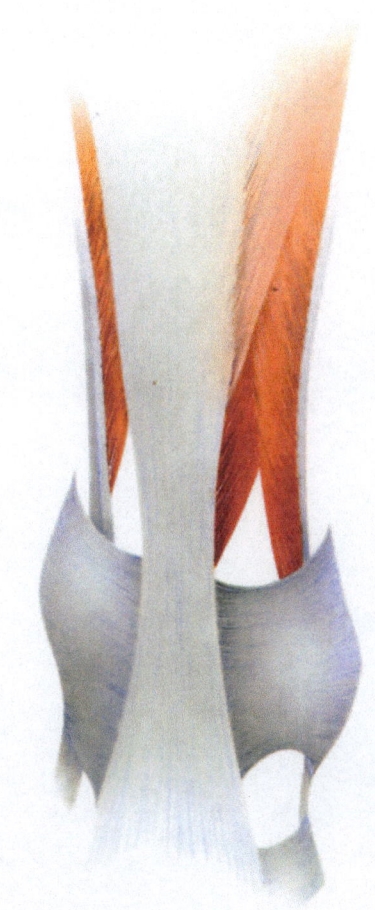

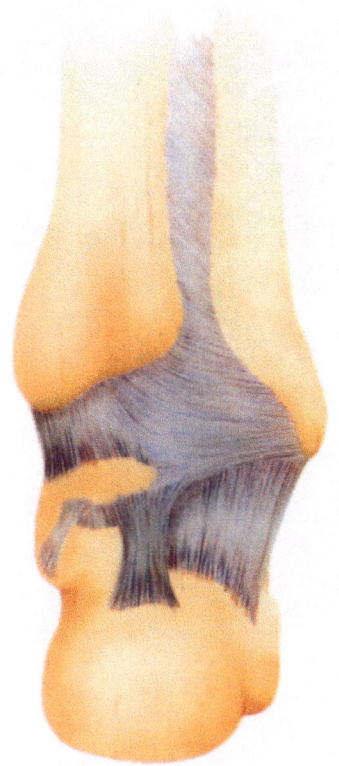

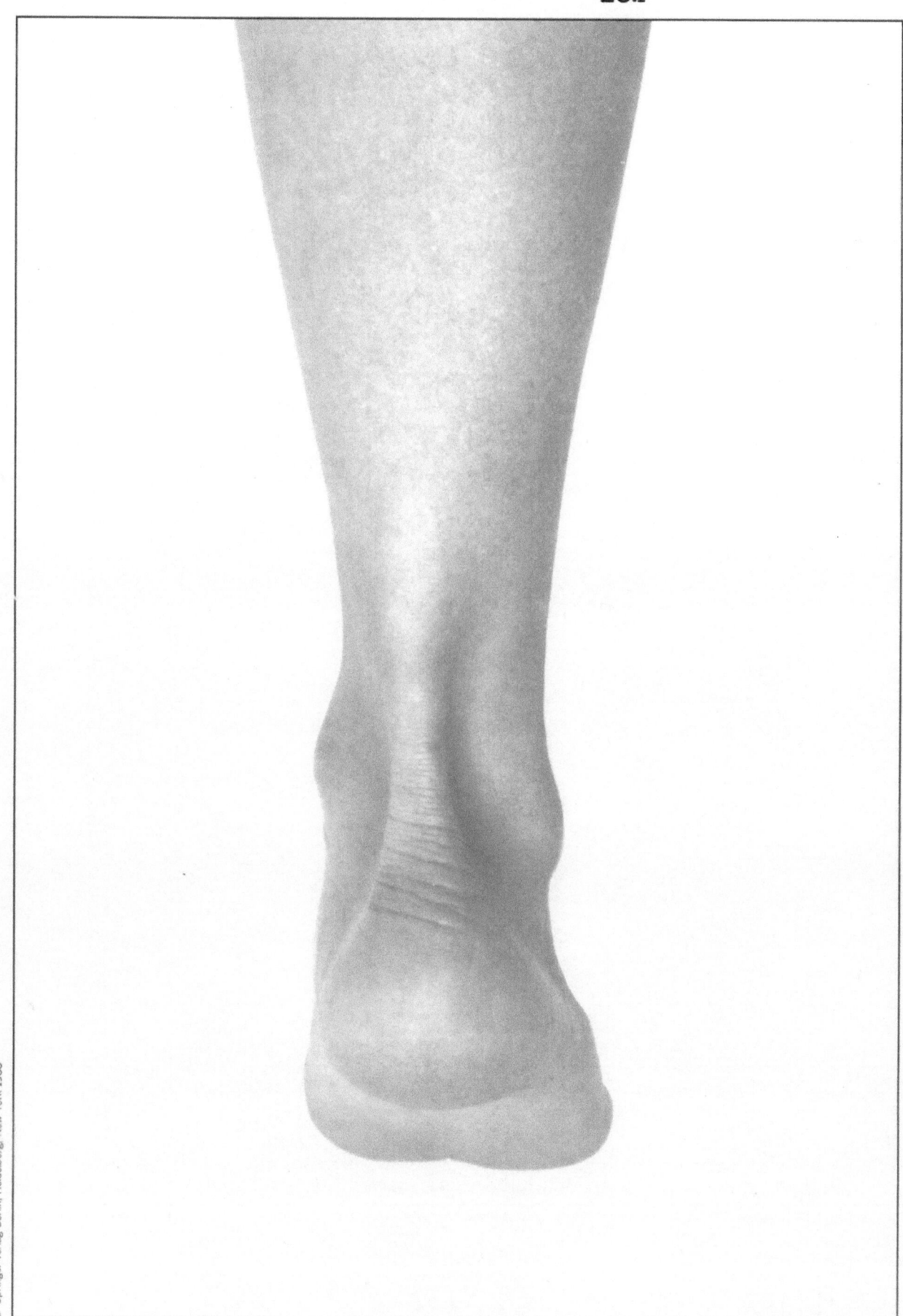

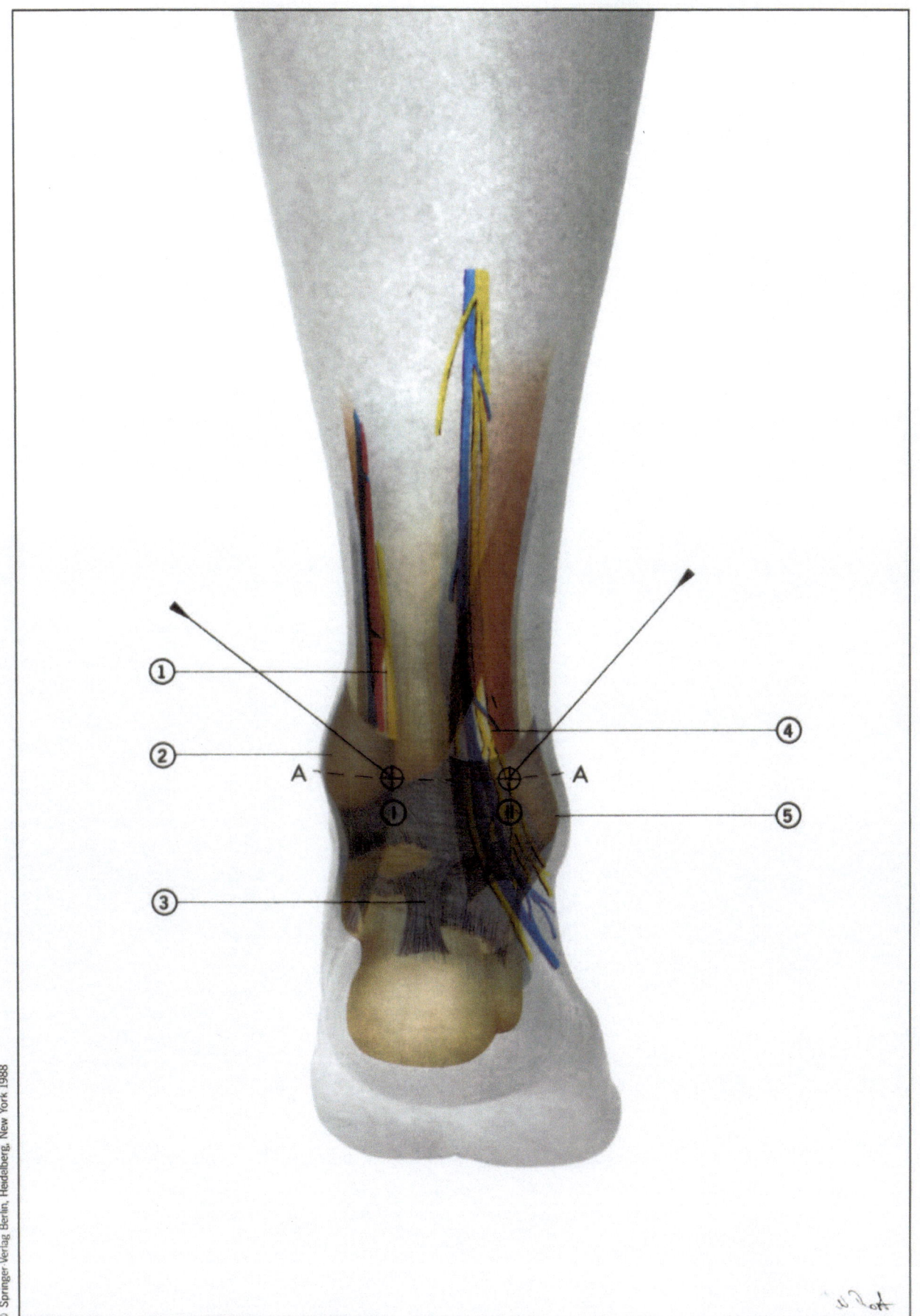

Ⓘ Injection site for tibial nerve block at the ankle. Ⓘ Injection site for sural nerve block at the ankle. A - - - - A: Line along which skin infiltration is carried out. ① Tibial nerve (alongside posterior tibial artery). ② Medial malleolus. ③ Flexor retinaculum ④ Sural nerve. ⑤ Lateral malleolus